LIFE AND DEATH iN KOLOFATA

D1569570

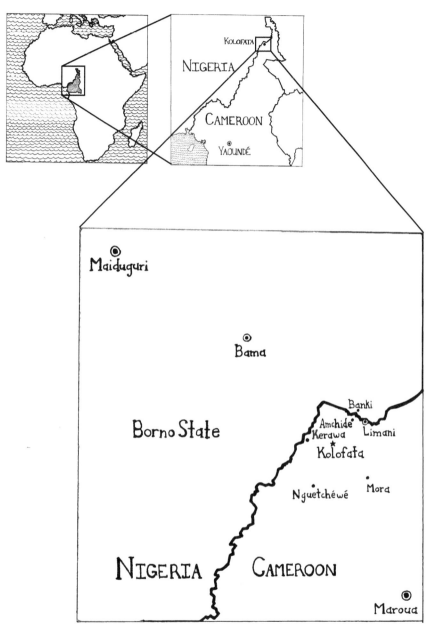

Map by Audrey Randall.

LiFE AND DEATH iN KOLOFATA

AN AMERiCAN DOCTOR iN AFRiCA

ELLEN EiNTERZ

INDIANA UNIVERSITY PRESS

This book is a publication of

Indiana University Press
Office of Scholarly Publishing
Herman B Wells Library 350
1320 East 10th Street
Bloomington, Indiana 47405 USA

iupress.indiana.edu

⊗ The paper used in this publication
meets the minimum requirements of
the American National Standard for
Information Sciences—Permanence
of Paper for Printed Library Materials,
ANSI Z39.48–1992.

Manufactured in the United States of
America

Cataloging information is available from
the Library of Congress.

978-0-253-03237-9 (cloth)
978-0-253-03238-6 (paper)
978-0-253-03239-3 (ebook)

1 2 3 4 5   23 22 21 20 19 18

This book is dedicated to the mothers and children of Africa.

It is reserved only for God and angels to be lookers on.

Francis Bacon

Contents

Acknowledgments

MANY YEARS AGO, Dan Carpenter, then a columnist for the *Indianapolis Star*, got hold of letters I had written to my family from Cameroon and suggested that a book be made of them. When I finally had time to do this, he was the first person I approached for criticism and guidance. For his inspiration, wisdom, and perseverance I am humbly grateful.

At the age of seventy-two, my mother bought a computer and taught herself to use it. She started typing the hand-written letters I sent from Africa and collecting them in a file so that when the day came, as she presumed it would, when I wanted to do something with them, I would have that huge step already out of the way. Without her hundreds of hours of tedious transcription, I'm not sure I would have had the pluck to begin. While I was in Africa, she wrote to me daily on sheets of thin white notepaper—a different color ink for each day of the week—that she folded into a plain number 6 envelope every Monday morning. I cherished the image of her walking to the sidewalk outside their home every Monday, slipping that envelope into the black mailbox, and then lifting the red flag to signal to the mailman that there was something to pick up. Her letters to me were my incentive to write back, and this book is as much hers as it is mine.

My father died before he could see it, but he would have been pleased, I think, that it got done. My love of writing comes from him.

My twelve siblings—Fran Einterz, Bob Einterz, George Einterz, Diana Einterz, Cora Randall, Mike Einterz, Anne Lewandowski, Nancy Woolf, Theresa Willard, Andy Einterz, Katey Einterz Owen, and Johanna Webber—supported me in a million ways throughout my time in Cameroon and in other countries before that, and I thank them for the strength of their devotion and the warmth of their embrace. For many years, several among them and their children have quietly contributed substantial funds to further health care and education in Kolofata.

From the beginning, the people of Saint Matthew Parish in Indianapolis made sure we had what we needed to move on to the next step. They have been my lodestar.

Jackie French, Bev Richey, David and Sherry Abney, Judy Hipskind, Patsy and the late Tom Wisler, Marie Carson, Sue and the late Marty Moore, the late Joe Quill, the late Pauline Chelle, Sue Leonard, Craig and Lee Doyle, Michael and the late Pat Fisher, Jeanne Malad, Marilyn and Bob Hunter, Tom and the late Betty Herold, David Noyes, Karen and Bob Tarver, and others whose names would fill another chapter have given repeatedly of their time and treasure. I thank them all, and I thank the many who call themselves Anonymous.

Canada's Volunteer International Christian Service kept Myra and me fed for twenty-four years while ensuring that we were never alone in the challenges we faced in the field. It was always motivating to realize that ours were among the hands that embodied the VICS activist spirit of peace.

Fran Quigley and Gene Stone agreed, with apparent good cheer, to read my original manuscript, and I am grateful to them both for the gift of their time, care, and valuable comments. Thanks also to Rob Smith, Neil Sagebiel, the editors of Indiana University Press, and Bill Schneider for their interest and wise counsel.

Dr. Ken Flegel, a gifted physician, teacher, and friend, connected me to my first patients in Africa, and for that I will be forever in his debt.

Dr. Fabien Taieb brought laughter, bright ideas, and exquisite French cheese to Kolofata at times when I needed them most. I raise a special glass to him.

To my many students from around the world, thank you for all you taught me.

With his encouraging smile and a kind word, Dr. Baba Malloum Ousman reached out and caught me any time I started to falter, and Amadou Ali, my wise and omnipresent angel, brought light to every darkness. He kept me safe. I suspect I owe my life to him.

Myra Bates has been my dearest friend for longer than either of us cares to remember. In so many ways, she shouldered the heavier burden in Kolofata, and her courage, determination, and love made flowers bloom in the desert.

Finally, I am grateful to the people of Kolofata and its surrounding villages, to the staff of the Kolofata hospital, and to the hundreds of thousands of patients who placed their trust in us. They are the heroes of this story.

Author's Note

THIS IS A work of nonfiction. Letters excerpted are selected from thousands of pages written in Cameroon—all pen on paper and with the salutation "Dear Everyone" unless otherwise stated—and sent to my family in the United States. To improve clarity in some instances, punctuation and paragraph divisions have been modified, spelling corrected and superfluous words removed. Any other alterations or additions to the letters as originally written are indicated by square brackets.

"Muslim" and "Quran" have been employed throughout to accord with current English spelling.

Some names have been changed.

LIFE AND DEATH IN KOLOFATA

Part I

WHEN AT LAST they came for us, we were not there. There were over two hundred of them, dressed in baggy trousers and unbuttoned camouflage shirts over singlets smudged with dirt and drenched with sweat. They rode into town aboard white Toyota pickup trucks and Chinese motorcycles, and they brandished rocket launchers, RPGs, and AK47s. It was a predawn Sunday: July 27, 2014, the last day of the holy month of Ramadan.

Friends later described to us what happened. Screaming, *"Allahu akbar!"* over and over again and firing into the air, they shouted orders and demanded in Hausa, Kanuri, and broken English: "Where is Amadou Ali? Where are the American doctors?"

Myra and I, the American doctors (though Myra was neither American nor a doctor), had been living under military guard for fifteen months, going little more than from house to hospital, hospital to house, always with an armed escort. Boko Haram, the terrorist organization whose name in local parlance meant "Western education is sin," had been successively kidnapping foreigners from our part of northern Cameroon—a French family of seven, a French priest, a Canadian nun, two Italian priests, ten Chinese road workers—and we had known for a long time that we were on their list.

As it happened, Amadou Ali, a native son of Kolofata who by this time was Cameroon's vice prime minister, was still traveling up from the capital, Yaoundé, for the holiday. His wife, twenty-year-old son, and extended family members had preceded him and arrived in Kolofata the night before. Myra and I had recently departed for our biennial visit to our families in North America.

The attackers fired their automatic rifles into our Land Rover, our house, and the detached storeroom in which we had planned to hide should such a day ever come. Several of the men shouted that they should go to the hospital and look for us there. Others objected, and in the end they did not go. Instead they grabbed ten members of Amadou Ali's family and household, our canton chief, the chief's wife, and five of his six children, and they shoved their prey into pickups and other four-wheel-drive vehicles parked in the compound. Two soldiers, eight townspeople, and seven members of Ali's family and household who had tried to stop the abductions or who otherwise got in the way were killed. Bullets to the head, knives to the throat. The assailants then ransacked the rest of the compound's buildings before launching grenades into them and burning them and their remaining occupants to cinders.

Outside the compound the invaders gleefully sprayed rounds at random, pockmarking homes, electricity poles, schools, trees, signs, and people, and by the time they left, four hours after they had arrived, our peaceful little town was a bloody battlefield of smoldering buildings, dead bodies, and unspeakable grief.

You Will Also Require an Umbrella

WHAT I REMEMBER most vividly about the first time I ducked out of a plane newly landed in Africa was the heat that clapped its arms around me in a grip tighter than a lover's embrace. The scent of burning wood, kerosene, palm oil, and sweat permeated the air, and with a mix of fear and gratitude I drew it in with deep breaths. I was in Niamey, Niger, and this was June 1974. A village called Gouré, a thousand barren kilometers east of Niamey, would be my eventual end point. I was a Peace Corps volunteer and at nineteen had come to teach English as a foreign language to secondary school students barely younger than I. I did not know it then, and I would have scoffed had anyone suggested it, but Africa would continue to be my home or destination for the next forty years.

The second child and first daughter of Frank and Cora Einterz, I grew up in a raucous household, one of thirteen children. My youngest sibling, Johanna, was born after I was already in Niger. My parents stressed the importance of discipline and education, and like most of my brothers and sisters I worked hard and did well in school, sports, and a medley of other activities. By the time I graduated from college, though, I was impatient for my efforts to yield something more meaningful than a grade on a test or a medal at a meet.

My Catholic upbringing contributed to that, but so had John F. Kennedy, handsome and eloquent, when he created the Peace Corps and said that volunteers would be sharing in the task of bringing freedom and peace to the world.

In Gouré I enjoyed teaching, but I sensed that I was not inventive or engaging enough to be an outstanding teacher, and the moments of fulfillment seemed too few and far between. I looked around my dusty, dingy village, at the skinny mothers, potbellied toddlers, and scrappy-haired children with running sores, and I thought about becoming a doctor. I would serve in this very place, or in some place much like it, where a little help might relieve a great deal of pain and every patient had a story to tell.

I started medical school at McGill University in 1978. Halfway through, I decided it would be smart to make sure that being a doctor in a poor, hot, underdeveloped setting was still what I wanted to do, so I arranged to spend three months with Our Lady's Missionaries, a Canadian community of nuns who ran a primary care clinic in rural Nigeria. It was a difficult summer, but the experience of living among and serving the poor only increased my desire exponentially.

After graduation and a twelve-month mixed internship in medicine and surgery at Montreal's Royal Victoria Hospital, I joined a Catholic parish run by an Irish Holy Ghost priest in Naka, Nigeria. For the next six years I directed and developed what would become the parish's fifty-bed clinic and orphanage.

The two superb Irish nurses with whom I worked in Naka returned home in 1986, and their departure left the clinic with no one to take charge of day-to-day administration. I asked a Canadian friend from college, Myra Bates, if she would consider taking the job. It was an outlandish proposal, and she treated it as such, but a little wrangling and cajoling convinced her to come for a visit. After that visit she took a leave of absence from her job in Montreal, signed on for a year, and then ended up staying for two more. We both left Naka in 1989 to pursue advanced degrees in public health at Tulane University's School of Public Health and Tropical Medicine in New Orleans.

While there, we searched the globe for a new posting, setting two criteria for determining our selection: the community had to have a real and unmet need for a doctor, and it had to be able to provide housing, since we knew we would not be making much money. We were offered jobs in Haiti, the Dominican Republic, and Sudan, but the first two sites seemed insufficiently needy and the last one too dangerous.

A Cameroonian classmate at Tulane, Dr. Kollo Basile, told us about a place called Kolofata in the Far North of his country. He explained that even Cameroonians thought Kolofata, isolated and exceedingly poor, was the back of beyond, and few wanted to work there. Civil servants who had caused trouble elsewhere were posted to Kolofata as punishment. Schools were generally scorned. Languages were multiple. Daytime temperatures during the three-month hot season hovered around 115 degrees in the shade. Children were unvaccinated. Exotic tropical diseases and the diseases of poverty were abundant. The district had no paved roads, no electricity or running water, no telephone or post office, no hospital, no doctor. I told Kollo it sounded great.

But, Kollo said, it is not enough to be in an area of need, even with the best intentions: you will also require an umbrella. He meant an umbrella of the political sort. You cannot go to Cameroon without an umbrella, he said, for the political climate there is prone to wayward, unpredictable storms.

As it happened, a man named Amadou Ali was from Kolofata, and Kollo felt he was just the person to ask. Head of Cameroon's Gendarmerie Nationale, Ali held the rank of minister in the government and, unlike other men from remote rural towns who had succeeded in school and happily shed the shackles of village life, Ali held his hometown close to his heart and worked constantly to improve the quality of life for the people there. Kollo knew him from his own time working as a young doctor in the Far North.

One morning Kollo arrived in class red-eyed and nubbly-haired, and I asked him what was wrong. He pulled out a single sheet of paper that he had filled with a letter written longhand. It began, *"Excellence, bonjour!"* and it described the offer made by two classmates, one a doctor, one a specialist in international health, to work in an underserved area in Africa or elsewhere, provided the destination was one of true need where housing could be offered by the community. He suggested that Kolofata might fulfill the requirements. He also mentioned the umbrella.

To get the wording right, Kollo said, he had been up all night. We checked the letter and found no fault. He folded it, placed it in a stamped envelope, and dropped it in the mail.

It took almost two months for a reply to come, also through the mail. Amadou Ali assured Kollo that he had a small guesthouse on his compound in Kolofata that could be put at the disposal of the medical team, and he would contact the minister of health in Yaoundé and the American ambassador to Cameroon to procure an official invitation and establish other formalities as needed. In other words, he would be happy to be our umbrella.

For our part, we contacted Brother Fred Sherrer, a missionary friend from Naka, who put us in touch with Father Dermot Doran, a Spiritan priest who had worked in Nigeria before returning to Canada to direct Volunteer International Christian Service, an ecumenical organization that sponsored volunteers in response to requests for help from parishes and institutions in Africa, Asia, and South America. We asked Father Doran if VICS would sponsor Myra and me in Cameroon and, on the strength of Brother Fred's recommendation and with little hesitation or fanfare, he said yes. We would be sent $250 a month to live on and a one-way ticket, the return of which would be provided after two years. That was the start.

To the End of the Earth

MYRA AND I arrived in Yaoundé on October 6, 1990, and reached Kolofata, a thousand kilometers to the north, three days after that. We made the trip up-country by plane to Maroua, the capital of the Far North, which was as far as a plane could take us, and then overland to Kolofata by way of Mora in the company of Dr. Baba Malloum Ousman, a veterinarian who worked in the Ministry of Livestock and Fisheries in Maroua. A native of Kolofata and a cousin of Amadou Ali, Dr. Baba was short and spry, with the dark skin and deep facial scars of the Kanuri tribe. We found his ready smile appealing and reassuring.

The landscape in the Far North was breathtaking. Night was falling fast when we left Maroua for Mora, but there was still enough crepuscular glow for us to see the geologic eruptions that flanked the road on either side. It was as if we were riding along the bottom of a sea after all the water had evaporated. Some of the hills were terraced and farmed in variegated patches. Others were just rocks, smooth giant boulders mounded one on top of the other and reaching up a hundred meters or more to the sky. They looked precarious, as though a simple nudge could set off an avalanche and boulder after boulder would come tumbling down. Against the base of the hills, small villages were nestled, their inhabitants evidently convinced that the rocks towering above them would never budge.

The road leading northwest from Mora to Kolofata was only twenty miles long, but it took us an hour to get from one end to the other. The rainy season had cut deep gashes along its tracks, and trucks lumbering back and forth had deepened the ruts, widened them, and mounded up their edges. The going was slow, the night black, the air stiflingly hot, and Myra and I wondered aloud how much farther away the end of the earth could possibly be.

Not much, as it turned out at last. "This is Kolofata!" Dr. Baba exclaimed joyfully, and we had to take his word for it, for we could make out nothing in the night outside the Peugeot's windows. It was not until we entered Amadou Ali's compound that we realized Kolofata, or this compound at least, had some sort of electricity. No other house in town had been lit.

Dr. Baba took us directly to the house made available for our use, and we settled in the sitting room around a wooden coffee table. Myra and I sat on the couch. Dr. Baba sat opposite us in an armchair, and half an hour after our arrival, a young man in blue jeans and a red sleeveless t-shirt appeared at the door. Dr. Baba stood up, extended his hand in greeting, and ushered Dr. Marc into the room. This was the freshly graduated Cameroonian doctor we had learned about only after our arrival in Yaoundé. He was from the South and had not asked to be posted to Kolofata. No one asked to be posted to Kolofata. We shook hands, expressed mutual delight. He welcomed us, inquired about our journey, told us we would be a breath of fresh air as he was swamped, there was much work to be done, and the people here were not easy. I thanked him for his cordiality. We talked weather, roads, food. I asked him which of Kolofata's languages he thought we should start learning first. "Oh no," he replied, "no need for that. You can always get someone to translate for you."

A man dressed in white pants and white safari shirt came into the sitting room from the back door and set a tray holding two enamel pots, a pile of glass plates, and soup spoons on the coffee table. Dr. Baba introduced him as Moussa, Monsieur Ali's housekeeper and cook. A small boy came behind him with a second tray holding glasses and bottles of Fanta Orange and Coca-Cola. Moussa pulled a bottle opener from his pocket and served each of us a drink while we helped ourselves to plates of steaming rice and spicy red sauce laden with onions and chunks of beef.

It was hot enough in the enclosed little house for sweat to be trickling down our cheeks and arms. Crickets—hundreds of them—bounced off floors, walls, and furniture. The smell of fresh paint hovered above the stew.

Conversation remained perfunctory—the heat, our journey, the hospital such as it was. Dr. Marc said he would be showing us around in the morning, but then he would be leaving for a few days to visit friends on the other side of Maroua.

After the men left, Myra and I did our best to wash the dust of the road off our bodies before falling into our beds and sweating through the night. In the morning Dr. Marc met us at the front gate and accompanied us on the walk up to the hospital.

It consisted of three small concrete buildings, each with a few cramped rooms. The largest building, fifty feet by thirty feet, was set along the main laterite road that cut through Kolofata's southern edge and ended, six miles to the west, in Nigeria. The building held a room with four cots, a cubical that served as the delivery room, another that had a microscope and staining trays on the cement counter, two tiny offices, and a closet identified as the operating room.

"I have done four Caesarian sections already," Dr. Marc proudly explained. "Of course," he added, giving me a knowing nudge, "they were not really necessary." I looked at him, felt alarm, forced a smile.

Of the other two buildings, one was a third the size of the first and had a room with two cots, an office, and a storeroom. The smaller building was roofless and unused.

On that first morning, three patients were hospitalized in the main building. All were children receiving perfusions of yellow fluid.

As we stood in this ward, Dr. Marc, wearing a white coat over his jeans and the sleeveless shirt of the night before, introduced me to his staff: Nurse Emile, bushy-haired and sullen-eyed, wore a shirt unbuttoned to his navel. Nurse Joseph was chugging a bottle of Coca-Cola. A midwife named Aissatou was crouching in a corner and holding her head in both hands. Nurse Mohamed, sporting a Detroit Tigers baseball cap, carried a small black radio that hissed. He appeared to be flirting with another midwife, Iza, whose cheeks were scored with Kanuri scars. The sole native of Kolofata, Iza was also the only one of the staff who spoke any of Kolofata's local languages. She translated for everyone else.

Across the road was a two-room whitewashed building known as the pro-pharmacy. Scantily stocked, managed by the mayor and staffed by a nurse named Ousman, the pro-pharmacy was where inpatients and outpatients were sent to buy medicines prescribed by hospital personnel.

Walking in the sand around the building was hazardous. As I stepped gingerly amid discarded needles, dressings, and the like, I suggested to Marc that we might arrange a little cleanup session.

"We could," he agreed, "but then it would only get littered again."

He showed us the room he had cleared to be our office. There were not, he apologized, enough rooms for each of us to have an office. We assured him that was not a problem, and the room he gave us was big enough to fit two chairs on either end of a table and still have a chair for patients on the side. It occupied the northeast corner of the main building. Of its two glassless windows, one faced the laterite road as it approached Kolofata from the east and the other, in the north wall, faced the road as it passed parallel to the building.

Laterite is red earth rich in iron and aluminum. It is found in the tropics and is favored as a coating for dirt roads because during the rainy season it reduces the slipperiness of unadulterated black mud. During the dry season it is transformed by revolving tires into clouds of red dust.

Kolofata is six miles east of the border town of Kerawa, which has a Nigerian half and a Cameroonian half. Motorcycles, cars, trucks, and tankers going east to west or west to east between Kerawa, Nigeria, and anywhere in Cameroon have to pass through Kolofata, and this road beside our new office was the only one they could use. It took us one morning to discover the consequences. Motorcycles laden with cartons of goods, mufflerless cars, pickup trucks packed with passengers, lumbering lorries overstuffed with wood and sacks of onions and grain, and maroon tankers filled with fuel all roared by from dawn to dusk, and each one deposited its share of red dust and debris onto our table, chairs, clothes, hair, and skin, and with every breath the stuff seeped redly into our lungs.

In Yaoundé Amadou Ali had predicted that the instant we arrived at the hospital, people would swarm by the dozens to it. This did not happen. There were two principal groups who used the hospital: students from the local middle school and wives of civil servants. In general the civil servant wives who came looked more bored than sick, and the students just seemed happy to be out of school.

The workday for all public services was split in two, after the prevailing French model: 7:30 to 12:00 in the morning and 2:30 to 6:00 in the afternoon. Our house was a kilometer and a half from the hospital. We made the round-trip walk twice a day and used the time to meet and greet. Women sat by the side of the road selling fried bean cakes and plastic-wrapped packets of shelled peanuts. Men lolled on mats under trees in front of their homes. Children kicked stuffed socks and empty tomato paste cans in the road, raising dust and shrieking. They always stopped their game to let us pass. Every morning a three-year-old girl named Ashi ran out into our path and joyfully wrapped her arms around my legs.

So Here We Are

Sunday, 14 October 1990

Dear Everyone,

I will begin this letter as I imagine I will be beginning most of my letters, having no idea when it will finish or when a chance will come to post it. And as I'm sure will be the case many times again, it is difficult to know where to begin.

We left Yaoundé by plane on Friday afternoon, arrived in Maroua just under 2 hours later with a 20 minute stop in between. We were met in Maroua by a Toyota pick-up and stopped there and then in Mora to meet the necessary dignitaries, all of whom had known in advance of our arrival and were exceedingly gracious. On, then, to Kolofata, where we arrived at about 8:30 (darkness falls at 6:00).

Great effort had gone into preparing a nice place for us. Our little house had been newly painted, a new stove had been placed in the kitchen, which itself was newly tiled. The compound was immaculately clean, as was the house—cleaner, I fear, than it will be now for a long time. The house is very small, consisting of 3 rooms: a sitting room flanked by two bedrooms, each with a full bathroom attached. Each bedroom has a double bed and a wardrobe. Separate from the house in front is a large storeroom, and attached to that is a thatched rest area, lovely and cool. Separate from the house in back (15–20 yards away) is our kitchen. The floors in the house and kitchen are vinyl tile, the walls cement, the ceilings varnished plywood, the roof corrugated aluminum. There is running water which must be used sparingly and electricity—at least for the moment. We make up one corner of a huge compound which itself is enclosed by a wall. It is a very comfortable set-up.

Medically the place is really and truly, unbelievably pathetic.

We go there early Saturday morning. The grounds all around are strewn with old intravenous bags, needles jutting up from the sand, soaked bandages and cotton wool, crushed glass vials, discarded syringes, and papers, plastics and wrappings of every description. They lie like a broad moat all around the clinic, stretching over to the primary school next door. Inside there are dirty needles, syringes, tubing, bandages and tongue depressors scattered about on tables, beds, sinks and all over the floor. The cement walls are crumbling and unpainted, the ceilings are rust-stained and droop ominously, the mattresses are caked with dirt. Massive globs of cobwebs laden with bat droppings dangle from the ceilings and decorate the walls. A nurse, in trousers and a shirt seemingly unchanged for three or four weeks, leans against the foot of a bed, sipping from a Coke bottle. A child's throat is examined; the tongue depressor then is snapped in two and tossed on the floor. There is not an aspirin in the place—nor in the town. There are half a dozen different medicines, most of them useless, a couple potentially highly lethal. Administratively there is such a system of locked doors, checks and balances and divided responsibilities that it is inconceivable that an emergency could ever be handled. In fact it is difficult to think of any medical problem that can be handled.

The people know. They come 5 or 6 a day. They get a prescription. If they have money they go to the city 1½ hours away to fill it. If not, they throw it away and go home. First, though, they have to pay for the consultation ($2.50). A patient in serious condition is "admitted." There are no medicines with which to treat him, however, and he usually figures this out pretty quickly and disappears within a day.

The young doctor has been here since April. He seems to have the understanding and skills of a second year medical student, although he is not averse to practicing on willing subjects. Apparently also he is a hothead and occasionally strikes his patients, though I have yet to see this.

So here we are. This week we will be getting out into the surrounding villages to see what is going on and get a feel for where/what the needs are. Marc has no interest in anything more remote than Kolofata (which must be like a plunge into hell for him) so our best tactic may be to develop a healthy bush program while slowly, patiently trying to nudge home base into order.

Before leaving the United States, I had secured funding for the purchase of a Land Rover Defender 110 to be shipped from England. Monsieur Ali told us that while awaiting its arrival he would put his old Renault 12 at our disposal and send Bello Damna, one of the Yaoundé chauffeurs whose job was to run errands for Ali's wife, to Kolofata with us to drive it and maintain it.

The car was a beige station wagon that had rolled off the assembly line in 1970. The driver's side rear door could be opened only from the outside, the passenger's side front window could not be opened at all, and the floor in the back was rusted clear through. Passengers could see the ground pass under their feet as they rode, and at all times exhaust fumes mixed with dust wafted in. But the engine hummed, the wheels turned, and the car most days could get us from point A to point B.

Bello was thirty years old and married to Dasso, with whom he had a young son and daughter. He was a northerner but from a village four hundred kilometers south of Kolofata. Like most people from anywhere south of Kolofata, he considered himself naturally superior to Kolofatans and was quick to shake his head and cluck his tongue at their apparent refusal to better themselves.

He wore Western garb—button-down shirts and zip-up pants, no bonnet. A smoothness in his cheeks and over his joints hinted at a tendency to gain weight too easily, but in those early days he was fit, muscular, and strong. His skin was mahogany in hue, his complexion flawless.

He had been around cars all his life and believed he could fix anything that broke, and if it happened that he could not actually fix whatever it was, he could, by dint of brute force, make it work, at least for a while. He was fond of heavy hammers.

When it became clear that we were not going to reach the people of our district by sitting in the hospital choking on dust and waiting for them to throng to us, we decided to venture out of the hospital and go find them.

> *Thursday, 18th. We have just completed a tour of the district, spending four hot dusty days visiting 30 villages around Kolofata. I believe there are 10 or 15 more we may try to get to next week. We have met all the chiefs and indicated that we would be setting a day with each for the purpose of sitting with the people to talk about problems, needs and possibilities. All expressed words of welcome and pleasure with this and assured us of their full cooperation—we'll see, but anyway words of welcome are more promising than indifference or displeasure.*
>
> *The need for medicines and understanding among the health professionals of how to use them is acute. The government hospitals cannot serve the poor as they are now set up, and the poverty is wrenching. People barely eke out a living from the dust. Whole villages are populated by emaciated children and adults. A patient may scrape together enough money for a day or two's worth of treatment, but not a whole week's worth, let alone more. Prescriptions for useless medicines are doled out, and the ignorant sick have no way of knowing which are truly needed for cure and which are fluff.*
>
> *The hospitals can only be of service to the better off. In general people eschew "modern" medicine—perhaps because it has yet to prove itself of any greater value than herbs and roots.*
>
> *Language is a huge impasse. The situation is complicated, there being numerous tribes in the area, each with its own language. Sometimes people from neighboring villages a few kilometers apart are unable to communicate with each other. There are few if any native Fulfulde speakers, but nevertheless Fulfulde serves as a sort of shared language—although a given village may have only 1 person who can understand Fulfulde. A communication therefore may have to be passed from one translator to the next before arriving at the ear of the person addressed. I ask a question in French, the nurse translates into Fulfulde, a villager translates the Fulfulde into Kanuri, and then another may have to translate the Kanuri into Mandara or any of the other languages. I must become competent in Fulfulde, and I would like to get hold of enough Kanuri to get by. But given the situation, you can imagine an instruction is never given*

fewer than 3 times, and the asking and answering of a simple question can take a long time. I am amazed at how isolated the people have remained and at how different languages and cultures have remained intact with such short distances between them.

The roads are terrible. We suffered 2 flats in 4 days, both in brand new tires. At times we were cutting blindly through the bush, nowhere near anything that could be called a road, headed in the general direction in which we were told the next village lay. My little compass has been my constant companion and has served me well already! In the rainy season many villages are completely cut off, and I'm told even a Land Rover cannot reach them due to swollen rivers without bridges.

We have spent what little spare time we have had in setting up the house, and it is starting to feel like home. I like it.

Marc has been gone all week, so I've also been holding the fort at the hospital. Making early tentative moves towards getting the place cleaned up.

We have our work cut out for us. I wish our drugs were here.

We are both in great health. I have yet to start running, but soon. Hope you are well. Much much love, E

Every Day Someone's Child Dies

WE STARTED GOING to two or three villages a day. At each village we set up under a tree and spoke to anyone who would agree to talk to us. Myra received the women and children; I took the men. We asked a set of questions aimed at helping us understand how each village was structured, what its economic situation was, what problems the people felt they had, and what solutions they imagined for those problems. We tried to get a crude measure of infant and maternal mortality, nutritional status, and commonly held notions of sanitation and hygiene. In general conditions were dismal, though people had a knack for shrugging off the worst. When asked if he felt his village had any health problems, one old man replied, "Well, no, not really, but our food is running out, there will be no water left in our well by the end of the month, and when we are sick, there are no medicines." In another village the chief snorted, "Yesterday a child died. The day before two children died. Every day here someone's child dies." Then he added, as if to wonder whether the loss of one child a day was exceptional, or perhaps to excuse himself for having had the audacity to suggest that things might be otherwise, "But we are a big village." Big meant sixty families.

I was called to another village after five children died in two days, and the *sous-préfet*, the local representative of the federal government, wanted to know if an epidemic might be afoot. I questioned the families of the dead and determined that the children had died of different causes, not one disease running rampant. I took advantage of the visit to examine the town's sick children, all seventy-one of them. A hodgepodge of pus-dripping eyes and ears, skin sores, malarias, and respiratory tract infections occupied me for the day. Having come with few medicines, I made a list of names and ailments and told the parents that I would go into town and buy what I could at the government pharmacy and then, if they were willing to pay, bring the drugs back the next day. All agreed. The following morning, as each child's name was called, the father or mother stepped forward. When told the price of treatment, some simply shook their heads and turned away. Others paid to treat one but not the other of their children. Some whose children had two problems took medicine for only one, and parents of the sickest did not even bother to come. My heart was breaking to see any of this, knowing as I did that it need not be.

Myra and I worked hard to get the hospital looking less like a hazardous waste site. One of the things we discovered during our village outings was that people spoke bitterly against the kind of reception they received in the hospital, where, they said, they were treated like animals. It was hard for me to argue. The small staff were undisciplined, money was dubiously extracted from patients, and the poor were victims of experimentation. Needles were routinely used to inject twenty or thirty patients at a time without being sterilized. Uncooperative patients were physically abused. The medication a patient received was as likely as not to have anything in common with the medication ordered. A newborn taking his or her first breath of air was suctioned with a dirt-smeared suction half clogged with some other baby's blood and mucus.

I was not sure how things would progress at this "hospital" so clearly unworthy of the name. I was more certain of what might be accomplished in the villages, although I knew that whatever inroads we made would be rutted with frustrations.

A Canadian organization called GEMS arranged a shipment of medical supplies for us, and at the end of October we joyfully took reception of twenty-five parcels of such things as microscope slides, tape, bandages, and kidney dishes. We were still awaiting an order of drugs coming from Europe. In the meantime we borrowed a basket of ten different medicines from a mission clinic outside Mora. These included two antibiotics, an antimalarial, medicines against worms and amoebas, two kinds of analgesic, iron tablets, vitamins, and a topical lotion to treat scabies, and they were enough for us to start to treat a surprising number of ailments.

Once Myra and I had a picture in our minds and a rough map on paper, we began going out on a regular basis to selected villages to offer treatment for the sick, vaccinations, child weighings, antenatal visits, and health education talks. Some days we were kept busy from seven a.m. to seven p.m. Other days we spent most of our time sitting under trees, waiting for people to work up the nerve to come see us. There were days when we arrived, unpacked our boxes and bags, and sat the whole day under a tree without seeing a soul. In the afternoon on such days we packed everything back up, thanked the chief for his hospitality, and assured him we would return on the same day the following week. In time, even in these most skeptical villages people started gathering up their courage and venturing over to us. Usually the old people, bent with back pain and limping with bad joints, were the first to come. After submitting to our ministrations and consuming our medicines, they did not die, did not turn into frogs, did not explode or disappear. Some of them even got better, and from those fragile seeds, confidence and trust began slowly to take root.

We were happy to concentrate our efforts in the villages and were not keen on appearing too closely associated with the hated hospital. We still put in a few hours each day there and had to be satisfied with small victories such as the introduction, if not yet the adoption, of heretical notions like "First do no harm."

On the home front, we were comfortable. Power outages and water breakdowns were evidently going to be the source of constant irritation, so we stocked up on flashlights and batteries, and we kept plenty of buckets and jerricans filled at all times. Already we were becoming adept at taking a shower from a cup.

Since little French was spoken by anyone except civil servants, competence in at least one or two of the local languages was going to be critical if I hoped to be any good at doctoring. We enlisted a middle school boy named Chetima to come to our house once a week to teach us. Kanuri was our main focus, but we also had him teach us some Mandara and Fulfulde. Myra and I planned the lessons, and Chetima, who was fluent in all three as well as in French, taught us what we wanted to learn. Everywhere I went I carried a little notebook in my pocket, and people at the market, men lounging in the streets, and women in the compounds all delighted in teaching us new words and expressions. Pulling out my notebook and pen and writing down whatever they were trying to impart inevitably elicited gales of laughter. They raised up outstretched hands and slapped their knees and loved it.

Since coming to Kolofata we had often admired a small abandoned gray and yellow building that sat on the crest of a hill at the western edge of town. We did not know the story behind it but assumed some wealthy man had built it as a home and then decided not to occupy it. We were chatting one day with Amadou Ali's father when he asked us if we had come to Kolofata to take over the new hospital. We asked him what he meant, and he told us about the abandoned building on the hill. We learned that it had been built in 1986 by the Ministry of Public Health as a maternity and first structure of what was supposed to have become a full hospital on the site. Financial crisis struck, the plan was abandoned, and the nearly-finished building was left to the elements, which meant hordes of bats, lizards, and termites.

We decided to go up and take a look. The building was surrounded on all sides by thickets of burrs, so just getting to it required no small sacrifice. Once arrived at the front door we had to spend an hour picking spiny pods from our dresses, slips, flip-flops, and skin. For days afterward my thumb and index tips would be speckled red. Of the building's interior, much had been destroyed. A door and four cupboards had been devoured by termites, the stained ceiling indicated a seriously leaky roof, and layers of dirt covered the floors and walls. Token equipment—mostly beds and side tables—were rusted through. But the underlying structure of the cement-block building looked good. There were two small rooms and one larger one. One of the smaller rooms had ceramic tiles paving the floor and the bottom halves of the walls. The outside doors were undamaged metal, and of the three wooden inside doors, only one had succumbed to termites. There was no source of water or electricity, but the builder had planned for both: the tiled room had a double aluminum sink, and fluorescent tubes in fixtures lined the ceilings in all three.

As we looked it over, Myra and I were thinking the same thing—that at the very least something better could be made of this building. It could serve as a fine base for the programs we wanted to undertake and in time be the start of a new hospital. In my mind's eye the picture was clear as day: I could see the place cleaned up and decked in colorful posters, women sitting with children on benches and mats, a nutrition demonstration happening in one corner, well-child checkups in another. I could see training and periodic retraining sessions for community health workers, a small lab, a pharmacy, maybe even someday simple structures for rehabilitation and isolation. I could see many things, all good and wonderful and possible if we could get permission to work here. Enthusiasm and hope propelled us forward.

Then came a setback. In November a French ophthalmologist and his assistant arrived in town to offer free examinations and treatment of eye problems. Even in the short time I had been in Kolofata, I had become aware of the hyperendemicity of trachoma, a chronic and often blinding bacterial infection of the eye that requires medical and sometimes surgical treatment. The ophthalmology team should have been met by a multitude of patients, for in addition to those with other eye conditions, thousands had trachoma. Instead, the team was greeted by only eight people the first day, four the second. Asking around to find out why more were not coming, we learned that a rumor had filtered up from the south about foreigners traveling the country administering shots that were touted as vaccinations but were in reality designed to sterilize or even kill women and children. It was unusual to see white people in Kolofata, and residents immediately suspected these French newcomers of being the vaccinator-killers. Word spread, and at the end of their second day, the *sous-préfet* got nervous enough to summon the two humanitarians to his office and order them to leave his jurisdiction before the uneasy populace turned hostile. The team returned to Maroua, confused by the turn of events and wounded that their excellent intentions and goodwill had been so badly misinterpreted.

As the week progressed, it became clear that the problem was not going to disappear with the departure of the eye doctors. The rumors were a nationwide phenomenon that overnight arrested public health activities, especially immunizations and maternal/child health work, throughout the country. Even more than before, people around Kolofata started to flee and hide themselves at the first sound of an approaching vehicle. One of our nurses had a shotgun aimed at him as he rode his motorbike through a village. In bigger towns and cities, parents armed with farming implements and saws yanked their children out of schools. In quieter places like Kolofata, schools simply closed. Elsewhere, missionaries who had been working faithfully, competently, and trustworthily in primary health care for ten or twenty years suddenly found their clinics unattended.

A common belief was that politicians had started the rumors. For months newspapers had been filled with demands for the institution of a multiparty system, and many felt that anything that might be done to destabilize any part of the government must be a good thing.

Simultaneously, the government, encouraged by outside donors, had decided to embark on an aggressive family planning campaign, and for a week prior to the onset of the panic, Cameroon's media had been overloaded with items encouraging women to go to their health centers to ask for Depo-Provera, an injectable form of birth control. These articles often emphasized the difficulties of feeding increasing numbers of people. Ordinary folk, putting one and one together, concluded that the government was trying to eradicate poverty by eradicating the poor, or by at least rendering the poor infertile, especially now that the latest harvest had been so bad. People were divided on whether the injection killed or only sterilized, but in this case few distinguished a birth control shot from a measles vaccination. Any injection being promoted by the government was considered ill-intentioned and harmful. The more health workers tried to convince people otherwise, the more people were convinced instead that authorities of all kinds were in cahoots and that others, and especially the poor, were on their own against them.

The progress we had started to make in the villages was obliterated by this imbroglio. Doors slammed against us; women and children dropped their basins and bowls as they ran for their lives into the bush. Village men refused to allow their women to come near us. With two exceptions, village chiefs continued to meet with us, but I sensed it was not without a considerable bucking up of courage first.

We were not happy to be rejected, but we weren't discouraged either. A heavy woolen blanket woven of ignorance and isolation was wrapped so tightly and so suffocatingly around our district that the tiniest little tear, the tiniest little air hole, had to be seen as a sign of hope. The offer of a chicken, the recovery of a sick child, a village request for us to come back—such things kept us believing that better days were ahead.

Laying the Foundation

Friday, 14 December 1990

We are slowly and carefully, I think, laying the foundation of what I hope will be our work here. Two underlying uncertainties may rock it: one being the current nonfunctioning status of the "hospital" and the other being the ever-vulnerable population's exposure to the kinds of rumors that swept the country last month (and still linger). I am enclosing clippings from two Canadian papers about the genital theft rumors that resulted in riots throughout Nigeria, just to give another example of how absurd and extreme things can get when an ignorant population is stirred to believe the most ridiculous notions.

The hospital, as I told you, is in a state of limbo. The reasons are multiple but boil down to poor patient care and expense beyond the means of the majority of people. It would have to be radically overhauled operationally to be rendered worthwhile. In spite of its nonfunctionality, it Is, and as such it is part of The System, and it receives and generates reams of meaningless paperwork, and I think you would have to have been born a French African civil servant—code book in one hand, paycheck in the other—to fully comprehend the existential importance of that. It is not what a thing does that is significant, it is that it is. In this case it is tragic, for such resources as there are (which are by no means negligible) are squandered. And squandering begets squandering.

We have been told to develop our own programs in whatever way we see fit. So far the authorities have been nothing but supportive, as if saying, in effect, What we have tried has failed so go ahead and see what you can do. We have been given use of the building on the hill of which I wrote to you in one of my last letters. Last week the lizards and bats and termites were startled to a rude awakening in the form of two mask-wearing, broom-yielding, sponge-waving, pesticide-spraying white chicks.

Our intention is to turn the building into a primary health care center, where all aspects of the WHO gospel on primary health care can be applied, both preventive and curative services. Critical cases will still be managed in the hospital down below [at the other end of town]. We are working on regularizing our bush program, still plowing through the rubble left in the wake of the killer vaccine rumors, and are starting with eight villages which will be visited on a bi-weekly basis. Thus every morning we will be in bush, and every afternoon we will be in Kolofata. Going out should also give us a better idea of the epidemiology of diseases in the area, knowing which problems are of greatest concern when and where. And in the long run maybe people will be inspired to have a little more confidence in what the health services can do and what they have a right to expect when they seek health care. And maybe someday it will dawn on them that when they fall sick it is well within the realm of thinkable things that they should get themselves to the hospital for help.

So that more or less is where we are and where we think we are going. There is much work to be done, not just in terms of providing health care but in terms of opening minds—much the harder of the two to do, but no less fun. There is no precedent for the kinds of things we are doing and hoping to do, and being non-missionary missionaries working within the government system, we don't fit neatly into any of the code books. So we are blazing a trail of sorts, and for the moment at least the powers that be seem to be content to let us blaze where we will.

As for the respect of the local people—in Kolofata, I mean—I think we have that, but mostly due to our bumbling attempts to speak Kanuri with them. They just love it, and we go out of our way to take different streets when walking to work and to spend a few minutes greeting or chatting with someone and to shake all the grubby little [hands] of the hordes of kids who come running out after us shouting greetings in three or four languages. We go to market every Sunday whether we need anything or not and greet the grinning toothless old ladies and babble with them about nothing at all. People come to the house or up to the building or they stop us on the street or call us into their compounds to tell us their woes and aches and pains and occasionally to see someone who is seriously sick but has refused to go to the hospital because it is a costly, inhospitable place to go. I enjoy the people. For all the harsh misery of their lives there is something essential and pure and wonderful about them.

That is not to say that there are not also those who would rather we were not here—whether because we are foreigners or women or Christian or simply because we were brought here by a rich and powerful man and rich and power-ful men always have their enemies. Also the vaccine rumors, coming so soon after our arrival, did us no favor. But so it goes. One does not walk into a foreign culture and expect to be taken into the bosom of every household.

From our village visits we learned that about three-quarters of our local popu-lation were Muslims. The rest were Christians, both Protestant and Catholic, and animists. The area's non-Muslims were either civil servants temporarily posted to Kolofata from elsewhere in the country or else families that had migrated down to our plain from the hills around Kolofata.

Few Cameroonian Muslims had an inkling that there were multiple denomi-nations and branches of Islam. The notion of Sunni or Shia, Sufi or Salafi meant nothing to them. They were Muslim, members of the monotheistic religion of Abraham, and that was enough. They adhered to the five pillars—recitation of the creed ("There is no God but Allah, and Muḥammad is his prophet"), ritual prayer five times a day, almsgiving, fasting during the month of Ramadan, and pilgrimage if possible to Mecca for the hajj sometime before they died. They strove to accept that whatever happened was no more and no less than the will of God, and graceful submission to fate was therefore expected, violence against it abhorred.

Women of any age, education, or social status were chattel of men. The district's non-Muslims were considered by most of its Muslims to be inherently inferior.

19 December 1990

Dear Nancy and Harry [my sister and brother-in-law],

We are having a typical sort of beginning, with all kinds of ups and downs which leave us dejected one day and cheered the next.

If I were a Muslim woman I think I would simply aim the gun and pull the trigger to get the misery over with. (The question, however, would be which way to aim the gun.) Many of the "downs" we have experienced have been frustration over the inaccessibility of the women (and hence the children as well). In a conservative Muslim society, women are kept behind closed doors, never venturing forth from their compounds from one day to the next, possessing no money, having no right to make the most rudimentary of decisions, kept ignorant and illiterate. They live in total subservience to men and are required to go to extremes to demonstrate their submission—removing their shoes when they pass a man on a street, going down on their knees to either give to or receive from a man. These things render our work difficult, for one cannot hope to improve the health status of a population except through the women and children. This is not easily done when the women and children are locked behind closed doors or when it is of greater importance to spend scarce money to soothe a man's muscle aches than to cure a woman's kidney infection or a child's pussy ear. Thank goodness we ourselves are white—it seems to excuse our endless sins: going around with exposed heads and calves, keeping our flip-flops on at all times and our knees off the ground . . . What a terrible shame it is that men do not realize that by keeping women oppressed, they themselves are the ultimate losers. But such is the tragedy of oppression everywhere since the beginning of time, be it of women, blacks, Jews or any other group of people.

Life in general is good. Our mornings are spent in bush and the afternoons here in Kolofata. The people are very poor, and many of our villages consist of nothing more elaborate than huts made entirely of dried grass and millet stalks. These inside look remarkably like the drawings of the insides of caves, with stick beds and little piles of earth-colored pottery and utensils made of sticks and stones. All labor is done by hand—even the work of scarecrows is done by a boy who sits on a platform made of sticks at one end of the field and all day long shoos away birds. Only in the bigger villages can you find anyone who can read or write or speak anything except the local dialect. Water—or rather the lack of it—is a constant worry. Near as I can tell, most people, particularly the children, live in a state of almost continual ill-health which is more or less accepted as normal. So there is a great deal of work at many levels to be done, and I am curious to see how the new year will go.

Christmas Day 1990

Dear Everyone,

Just a note to tell you I am thinking of you.

The good news this week is that our drugs have arrived in Yaoundé and should be in Kolofata by Saturday. That is a relief. We are barely scraping by on our borrowed essentials. It will be nice to have a proper arsenal to work with again.

New Year's Day 1991. So the year has passed. We have had a busy week and were both laid low simultaneously by a respiratory tract infection that has hit scores of people—many progressing to pneumonia. The harmattan has begun in earnest. The dry cold wind howls and dust swirls and settles everywhere. The temperature has dropped as low as 73°, which I know makes you laugh, but for us that is wickedly cold. Little kids, barefoot, pantless, wearing only loose filthy smocks, stand outside their millet stalk huts and shiver. Their noses and ears and eyes all run and their faces are powdered white by the dust for which there is never enough water to wash. They cough and fuss and are bleary-eyed. They sleep at night huddled against smoldering fires that fill the hut with a grey smoke that stings the eyes and the nose and throat. It is probably difficult to comprehend the harmattan if you have not seen it, but remember the densest fog you have ever known and imagine it made up not of vapor but of dust—fine, fine dust so dense you can taste it. Run your hand through your hair and the smell of dust penetrates your fingers. Go for a walk and the dust coats your eyelashes white.

We were both hit hard by whatever has been going around, but for a doctor (who is trying to build a little confidence up among the people) to fall sick is poor advertisement, so we did our best to keep going full steam, though it was not much fun. We are round the bend now, feeling much better, delighted to have had today a holiday and relatively work-free.

Saturday 5th. I am already concerned that the drugs will not last us as long as I had hoped, and we will be getting our next order going within the coming week. Between bush in the morning and Kolofata in the afternoon/evening, we are now seeing 50 to 100 patients a day—exclusive of well children who come just to be weighed or vaccinated and pregnant women who come just to be checked.

In our border villages, we are seeing a fair number of patients from Nigeria, so word seems to be spreading.

During the day, women may leave their compounds only to fetch water. Otherwise they are cloistered. In some places even the water fetching must not be done during daylight hours. They wear veils, though not across their faces, and the head and back of the neck are covered at all times. In public the front of the neck is covered as well. Middle-aged and older women have teeth stained a bright orange-red from years of kola nut chewing. For beauty, the younger women dye the palms of their hands and soles of their feet black and paint selected teeth pink or red with nail polish. They also put dabs of nail polish on their cheeks and foreheads and often wear an earring in their nose on the side: a ring or a stud. The men usually wear light cotton pajama-like trousers with a loose smock top. The richer ones have massive robes of expensive material and embroidery of a design, extent and elaborateness indicative of status. Of the people I have seen on numerous occasions in the villages, from chief to lowliest peasant, very few have I seen dressed in anything but the outfit they were wearing at our first encounter. Shoes, if any, are usually flip-flops which have been broken and repaired repeatedly. These are always removed upon entering a hut or rest area.

Meals are taken from communal bowls by clumps of people, the women with the children, the men with the men, and never within sight of one another. The roads at dusk are lined with huddles of men, eight to ten crouched around their pots outside the compounds, eating, each scooping a handful of pounded millet and dipping it into thick slippery green sauce and flipping it deftly, not to spill a drop, from pot to mouth.

At night people sleep in their airy huts on mats, sometimes on low stick beds, with their fires and their animals—chickens, goats, sheep, sometimes even cattle, [all inside]. The animals help with the warmth, I guess, and [being inside] they are protected from thieves. Flies are fierce. Children live with them feeding on their eyes and nose and mouth and any sores they might have. If there is enough water for cooking and drinking, there is not enough for bathing and washing clothes. In many villages what water is to be had must be dug out daily from holes in the sand.

The people cultivate millet and cotton, and both crops were decimated this year by a rainy season that started too hard and ended too early. The cotton is sold to the government [actually, a parastatal], which buys it at ever-diminishing prices (there are no competitor buyers) and which taxes each bushel sold, producing the cash only months after the sale. The millet is kept as the year's food supply, and when this runs out people hire themselves out at 50¢ a day and sell their livestock to buy food for their families. The meat sellers have been having a grand time, buying animals for less and less every week, and the price of millet goes up as the sum fetched for an animal goes down.

Most people in the villages are so illiterate and innumerate, and so unaccustomed to trading with cash, that the simplest of financial transactions are beyond them. They cannot be told an amount owed, they must be shown the coins or the bills, and then they must accept on blind faith that you have not cheated them [in giving] them back change. Transportation is by foot, bicycle, donkey or horse—the horses I have seen are pathetic, scrawny things. There are usually a few motorcycles in the larger towns, and there are several cars among the government employees in Kolofata. A few of the villages have one-room school houses; most have not.

Every village has at least one mosque, though often this consists of nothing more than a two-foot high mud wall set along a 12' x 12' perimeter. (Having once made the gross error of stepping inside one of these unbuilt buildings—women of reproductive age being forbidden to enter so sacred a place—we have developed a keen eye for knowing exactly which type of unbuilt building is and is not a mosque!)

When we worked in the villages, we adapted ourselves to whatever welcome we might receive. Most people's homes had little furniture, and in some villages there were no chairs at all, so upturned mortars were all we might find for sitting or writing on. Such days could be backbreaking, but with our crowds growing steadily we were little concerned with comfort. By mid-January we had had our first hundred-plus patient day.

Gestures of acceptance meant the world to us. The men of one village repaired a road that had been particularly rough on our poor car. In another village they constructed a table—wobbly, crude, and much too low, but a table nevertheless—because the week before I had struggled the whole day trying to write on my lap. Everything they could find—roofing rivets, bicycle spokes, strips of metal from tin cans, recycled wooden struts—seemed to go into its making. The men had evidently been sitting around waiting for us, for when we arrived, one of them hoisted this table proudly over his head and carried it to us. The chief of the village where a few months earlier a nurse had had a shotgun aimed at him sent an envoy asking for forgiveness and requesting to be put on our program. The men of yet another village constructed a shelter of millet stalks so that their women could enjoy some privacy when we examined them. All these acts reassured us that we must be on the right track.

The lack of water was a perpetual problem for almost all our villages. There was no running water anywhere. Outside the rainy season, streams and ponds dried up, the water table sunk ever deeper, pumps broke down, and wells, already scarce, too often ran dry. Where possible, we worked with different government ministries to get broken pump parts replaced and promised wells dug, and while these efforts amounted to little more than drops in the proverbial bucket, they meant a lot to the people of the villages whose lives were directly touched by them.

Soon after the 1991 New Year holiday, a US Army major and an official from the American Embassy in Yaoundé came to visit. A decision had been made that the Cameroon and American militaries would work together to conduct a mass antimeningitis vaccination campaign in Kolofata, and the pair had come to scout the area and get a feel for what kind of reception they might expect. They were extremely nice and typically American in their bright, eager, can-do cheerfulness. Over a spaghetti dinner outside in our courtyard, we talked about what should be done in advance to make the event a success. By the end of the evening, neither Myra nor I was convinced that they heard our gentle but pointed warnings about how the Muslims of the rural North were likely to regard a mass vaccination campaign undertaken by foreigners, a term applied to anyone, whether white, black, or purple, who did not hail from within a ten-mile radius of Kolofata. We would all find out soon enough.

Who among Them Ever Heard of Descartes?

FOLLOWING IRAQ'S ATTEMPTED annexation of Kuwait and the passing of a UN Security Council resolution authorizing the use of force if Iraq refused to withdraw, an allied coalition led by the United States began a massive aerial bombardment of Iraq on January 17, 1991. As often as possible, we turned on the radio and tuned into the BBC to hear the latest, though we never did this without trepidation, fearing what terrible thing we might hear. A distant but gnawing anxiety was the undercurrent of my every waking—and, I sensed, sleeping—moment that January and February, and like everyone else in the world I just wished the fighting would come to a swift end.

With the arrival of our first shipment of drugs, we were more at ease treating a broader range of patients. The drugs were not expensive, and payment was expected, but no one was denied treatment. Spotting the poorest among our patients was seldom difficult. Even before they started to tell me about their pain, they would fish from under a fold of cloth a ratty piece of plastic tied with string. Unraveling this they would extract a few coppery coins. Their treatment, they would sternly instruct me, should not exceed this amount. Sometimes a handful of roasted peanuts or an orange or a guava would be handed over as well if the patient suspected that the coins were not enough. We absorbed the loss, but we were not above tacking a compensatory franc or two now and then onto the bills of wealthier merchants and civil servants.

Our hope was that in Kolofata poverty would never be a reason for someone not to seek health care. We knew that there were and would be plenty of other reasons.

Three men appeared on our doorstep at nine o'clock one night. A thirty-year-old woman in the village, they said, was having fever, vomiting, and diarrhea. Mother of six, the youngest two years old, she had been sick for the previous five days and was now, they believed, nearing the end. Their village was only ten kilometers away and on the main road between Kolofata and Mora. Dozens of cars, bikes, and motorcycles passed their house every day, and the village had horses as well. I was furious that for five days the men had done nothing to bring this woman to the hospital, and I asked them to explain why. "No means," was their reply, and this only infuriated me further, for if the three of them had means to come to me that night, they also had means to bring the woman four days earlier. I asked them what they wanted me to do now, and they said sheepishly that they wanted me to come see her in the village. And so I understood: this was a woman they did not allow to leave the compound, and for that principle they were willing to sacrifice her life.

With our hospital-in-a-bag, Myra and I set out for the village and found the woman lying on a mat on the ground in a dark, smoky hut. She was moaning.

Her body was on fire, her eyes were hauntingly sunken, and her lips were bloody and swollen, allegedly from a bang against the corrugated metal of the door. Her teeth were bone-dry. She had been vomiting incessantly and unable to keep down the smallest drop of water.

By flashlight I gave her two injections and placed an intravenous drip, hanging the bag from a cord stretched across the hut. I showed the men how to look after it and her, and after staying until I thought her breathing had settled somewhat, we left her in their care.

The next day before dawn we stopped in at their village on our way to our morning's destination. We found the men seemingly unmoved from where they had been when we left them, but the smiles on their faces told us everything we needed to know. Our patient, too, managed a faint smile. Her vomiting had stopped, the dehydration had diminished, her electrolytes had gotten themselves back into line, and—best of all—she was hungry and asking for porridge.

I again asked the men why they had not brought her to hospital. They shuffled their feet, looked down, and shrugged. "Next time," was all they offered.

The hospital was seldom patients' first choice for health care. There were many alternatives. For the more modern-minded, pills (of dubious composition and usually from China or India) were sold in market stalls. For the more traditional, itinerant medicine men wandered from village to village, their satchels replete with roots, powders, barks, and herbs. Most also carried a corked gallon glass jug filled with a brownish infusion in which chunks of dark vegetation floated. Most villages had a woman who attended other women during childbirth. Women could also be healers, though female healers did not set up in the market or leave their own villages, and usually they were more specialized than their male counterparts.

Akin to traditional practitioners were marabouts, teachers of the Quran who dabbled in spiritual and herbal healing. The Quran was often their primary tool. When a patient came to a marabout and explained his problem, the marabout, in exchange for a fee that might be cash, a chicken, or a bowl of grain, wrote a passage from the Quran on his board, washed the ink off the board into a clay pot, and then had the patient drink the curative, inky fluid. Alternatively, he might copy a verse on a scrap of paper, fold the paper into a tiny wad, and pack the wad into a leather pouch that he then sewed up and fixed to a cord for the patient to loop around his waist, neck, or arm. Most people had at least a few of these amulets hugging different parts of their bodies, and sometimes there were so many of various sizes and shapes strung so densely and in so many directions around their neck that it was not easy for me to get my stethoscope over their heart and lungs. Often, marabouts were also adept social workers. They had more understanding of humans' vulnerability than of their physiology, though, and although many put this understanding to helpful use, others used it to hone lucrative skills of charlatanism. In this they were not alone.

Having completed six years of primary school, Zara was one of the most educated of Kolofata's women. The quality of primary education in our part of Cameroon was such that after six years she was still illiterate and innumerate, but the fact that she had gone to school at all made her a leader in the community.

Myra and I came upon Zara one afternoon as we walked down from the clinic. Cradling her jaw in one hand, she barely smiled as she explained that her tooth had been hurting for a week. She finally went to a healer who put a paste into her mouth and told her to hold it there for a few seconds before spitting it out.

Zara reached into the folds of her *pagne* and pulled out a dirty scrap of plastic crumpled into a little ball. Carefully she opened this packet and held it out to us. Within were four larva, each about a centimeter and a half long. They looked like snipped bits of a pipe cleaner. "This," Zara declared triumphantly, "was what came out." Startled, wondering if she really believed these huge creatures had been burrowed under her tooth, I searched her face for any sign of jocularity. There was none, only pain.

I asked her if she was feeling better now that the culprits were out. "Not yet," she said, groaning, pressing her hand more tightly to her jaw, "but soon."

Over the years we learned that this was a common technique of native healers. They were brilliant at finding ways to "remove" worms and insects from mouths and ears and assorted other apertures, much to the delight of their patients, who were thrilled to have tangible evidence of the cause of their malady. If after removal of the offending animal the malady still did not go away, then clearly, and through no fault of the healer, a witch had cast an evil spell, and other measures would have to be taken to counter the curse.

Another common treatment technique involved the firing of a glass bottle or animal horn and the immediate application of this hot instrument to the place of pain. This method was especially used for abdominal and chest complaints, so by the time they reached adulthood most people had numerous round patch-like marks over their abdomens, chests, and backs. Occasionally patients came with red, pussy lesions created when these burns became infected.

Knife or razor blade nicks inflicted by healers for the same reasons also were easily infected and had to be treated. Children were not exempt from this scarification treatment, and one of my earliest patients was a ten-day-old baby who had angry red welts two and three inches long all over his abdomen where the skin had been slit repeatedly to treat colic.

On our side of the medical divide, the stethoscope had its own magic, and I soon found that old people in particular were not satisfied if I did not use it long enough or in all the right places on them. They seemed to believe that it alone could cure a pain. Sometimes a patient would give me no peace until I had applied it from head to toe over every aching muscle and arthritic joint.

People had tremendous faith in their sorcerers, healers, marabouts, and quacks. This often defied what many would call reason, but as Dr. Baba, our veterinarian friend and cultural mentor, explained, "Who among them ever heard of Descartes?" Life and all its causes and consequences were perfectly logical. But their logic was not ours, their reason was not ours, and neither was their concept of what constitutes the universe. We only shared with them the struggle to make sense of it all.

In Their Most Dire Poverty We Find Wealth

Saturday, 16 February 1991

The week went by very fast. The weather is changing, heating up noticeably during the day, remaining more pleasant than cold at night. It is an interim period to be enjoyed, for in a couple of weeks the real heat, which so many people have warned us about, will be here.

We are also concerned about what the coming weeks/months will bring for the people as the stores from last year's meager harvest run out. Money is already short—even compared to what it was a month or two ago when the harvest was still new and people had some cash from their cotton crop. In spite of having sown as much as in previous years, those who did well harvested 10–20% of what they'd reaped the year before, and some ended up with nothing. People are selling their animals, others are scraping by as wood-cutters, collecting firewood to sell, others are borrowing from luckier relatives, others are hiring themselves out to wealthier farmers here and in Nigeria at a rate of 50 cents to $1.00 a day. There was talk a couple of months ago of a possible deal to get aid grain up from one of the big international agencies, but there has been no sign of that yet, and having seen such schemes in operation in both Niger and Nigeria, I would remain skeptical about it ever [reaching those in] greatest need.

Certainly along the fringes of society there are already signs of hunger. You should have seen our compound in the days after the [American] ambassador left. That Saturday there was a huge feast for her and the dozen or so other notables who were here for the anti-meningitis [vaccination] campaign. Under a thatched canopy at one end of the compound a massive table was set with bowls and platters overflowing with stews and sauces, vegetables, rice, yams, every kind of meat available, crates of drinks and for the infidels bottles of beer, wine and champagne. (One soldier, presumably knowing no better—or perhaps knowing full well—uncorked a bottle of Dom Perignon, let it foam out all over his fist and onto the Turkish carpets that had been laid on the sand, then lifted it to his lips and guzzled it like water, the whole bottle.) I suppose there were a couple hundred people there. There was more than enough food to feed all of them, and what was left got divided up among kitchen and house staff, relatives and neighbors. By evening the crowds had dispersed and the compound was again quiet but littered with bones, greasy mats and tables and bowls, stray spoons, empty bottles and in one corner, lost and alone, a pair of well-worn green and white flip-flops. Before nightfall, several men and young urchins of one of the poorer minority tribes slipped past the guard and made their way into the yard in front of our house. They proceeded to scavenge any remains they could find. They ran their fingers through the grease of discarded bowls, licking them clean. They upturned bottles of soft drink and beer, they dug through the sand, picking up bones and gnawing on them, they collected others in torn dirty plastic bags. Those who came that first day probably did pretty well. Others came the next day and again the day after that—still picking up bones in the sand, breaking them open and eating them—and eventually there was nothing more to be found.

Sunday, 17th . Last night a 45 year old widowed Mafa woman came to the house. She looked like so many of the Mafas—bonily thin, sunken, dressed in rags so threadbare and worn that all the colors look the same. (We have a 7 year old Mafa boy with a bad ulcer on one of his ankles whom we see every day for dressings. One day, when I was not going to be here the following day, I wanted to explain to him how to do the dressing at home. I had a Kanuri schoolboy in to help with translation. I told him to clean the sore and to soak his foot in a bucket of salt water and then to take a clean cloth—at which point the Kanuri schoolboy interrupted me abruptly and said, "These people don't have clean cloth," just trying to be helpful.) The woman was pained and short of breath, hot and hugging her ribs as if to stifle the pneumonia inside. She had been sick for a week. I asked her why she had not come earlier and she said she had no money, and it was only today that someone passing by saw she was sick and gave her ten naira—a dollar—which she now brought. I asked her what she ate, and she said millet, only millet, and of that only as much as she had money to buy in the market—a bowl now and then. Her own meager harvest had ended long ago, and the sun had burned all her cotton before it was ripe. To buy food now she depended on people passing by to give her a naira now and then. She had two children still alive, but both had left for Nigeria's greener pastures. I asked her how, since her harvest was so poor, she would have seed to plant again next year. She smiled for the first time and wondered aloud whether she would still be alive to have to worry about that.

The sick are so sick, the poor are so poor. And yet they never stop giving. We walk along the back roads of Kolofata and an old lady offers us a boiled sweet potato, insisting that we take and eat this delicacy. Another digs out a little wrapped bundle of roasted peanuts. Another hands us each a lime. A leper, whose chronic foot ulcer I dress every day, this week brought us a bag of five oranges, smiling with obvious delight as he handed them to us. None of them could easily afford to part with any of these things. But they seem to believe it is important to give, as if in defiance of their own deprivation, as if they know that in their most dire poverty we find wealth.

Tuesday, 26 February 1991

We are planning on going to Maroua on Friday, so if I am lucky I will get a chance to finish this before then. We had our first news of some sort of Iraqi withdrawal a few minutes ago. I hope it is truly the beginning of the end and if so I hope that what we do now we do right and with all wisdom and justice. I've a feeling that the hardest part, the part that will be the real determinant of success or failure, lies yet ahead.

Saturday at about five PM AA's gatekeeper, a thin man with a game leg, whose every sentence contains at least three different languages, came rushing to the house flapping his wings, saying a child was here, very sick, very serious, I must come. An entourage of five people entered the compound and on the back of one woman was a one year old child, his head and limbs hanging limp, his body heaving in rapid gasps, white foam bubbling out his nose and mouth. He was a pasty yellow color, his lips were cyanosed, and he was deeply comatose. One of the men was explaining that the child had ingested poison, a powdery granular substance used to kill the birds that destroy the millet. He was going on and on about how it had happened, how the mother had gone to bathe and the boy had been left in the care of older children. I stood there on the doorstep and looked at the froth pouring from the child's nose—I had never seen this except in the minutes preceding death; the heart fails, the lungs flood, the fluid overflows— and shook my head and flapped my own wings uselessly and said it was too late, it was too late, what could I do. The family remained firmly planted where they were, no one turning or moving or even crying. And so, I thought, I had better do something, and something must be everything until the child expired. So Myra and I shifted into high gear and turned our front step into an ICU and poison treatment center. We got some diuretic and steroid going into him and took a nasogastric tube and emptied his stomach and cleaned him out and flushed down some crushed [charcoal] tablets to mop up whatever poison might be left. [A] homemade suction device did a good job of keeping his airway clear. After this massive onslaught I was amazed that the little gaffer was still alive. He was only barely this side of the line, though—he was still in a deep coma, his color was ghastly, his chest was heaving, his heart was pumping out amazing acrobatic rhythms. We sat out there with him for several hours, trying to keep him hydrated, but not too hydrated, and his airway clear. Since he had not died when he was supposed to die, it seemed to me it might only be a question now of keeping him alive until the poison had been excreted or metabolized into nothing—unless of course the cardiac or brain damage had already been too great. After the initial flurry of activity was over, an old woman came rushing over and took the child from the mother's arms. She was Yatsoua, one of the town's traditional midwives, one of the old women with whom we used to spend our Saturdays sitting and talking under the trees when we first came to Kolofata. The child was her grandson, and once word had reached her about what had happened she had gone all over town looking for them. She was breathless and distraught. She just sat there on the ground, holding the limp baby, looking into his grey face, feeling his lifeless hands and feet. (Myra several times in between our ministrations kept commenting about what cute little feet he had.) She spoke his name over and over, "Brahim, Brahim," as if urging him to answer her. She shook her head and said to me, "We will go home." I looked at her and thought with great temptation how nice it would be not to witness the death of this child, but I said no, it would not be good yet to go home. I don't know if she mistrusted me or if she wanted to take the boy home to work her own magic on him or if she just wanted the family to be home and at peace, and the boy to be without tubes going into him, when he died. She complied reluctantly but without argument, and I did what little I could to gain her trust—speaking only in Kanuri, swabbing Brahim's eyes and face, keeping him clean and dignified and her as much as possible comfortable. She settled down and became an attentive partner in his care, helping me to suction him, turning him when I needed a different access. Every time I put a stethoscope to his chest or a light to his eyes or a finger to a reflex point she looked imploringly at me, and I knew she wanted me to say don't worry, it is better. And I wanted to say that, but fear kept me quiet, and we waited.

There were moments, when she held the child just so, when I thought his color was a little better, that his sunken dead eyes were a little fuller. A couple of times he gagged when I suctioned him—at least one reflex was working. But his pupils remained pinpoint, he reacted in no way to any other stimulus, his breathing was heavy and noisy.

The time came when there seemed to be nothing more to do but allow time to pass, and so I asked the family if they preferred to take Brahim and go sleep at home or if they would rather sleep here under our thatch shelter. They said they would go and come back first thing in the morning, and I said that would be good. Yatsoua lives only a few houses down, and that was where they would go. The mother tied him on her back and they all trooped out into the night, and I wondered if I would ever see the child again.

I slept fitfully and awoke early. Dawn came and there was no tap on the door. As the minutes passed I felt more dismal. We went out into the town in search of a lady selling little fried cakes—like donut holes—to which we often treat ourselves on a Sunday morning, and when we came back there was no one waiting for us. I guess our boy died, I stated the obvious, and Myra replied, You did all you could, which is her best and only reply when I start brooding over a failure, and I said, Maybe, but I'd kind of hoped that where I left off the good Lord would see fit to do whatever else had to be done. We sat down to our coffee and "donuts" and shortly were interrupted, as usual, by a patient seeking help. I was still talking to her in front of our kitchen when Yatsoua entered the compound. She was quiet and shy, but I called her [over] and greeted her. She was alone. Not wanting to ask, I gestured to inquire how things were. She smiled, bent both elbows and shook both fists. That means well. Health. Strength. Brahim? I asked. She smiled, bent both elbows and shook both fists. They were on the other side of the house, she said, pointing, and she said come see.

We went, and there they were, the mother sitting on our front step, the child in her arms. He was crying in bursts, squirming, whining, clearly in discomfort but very much alive. We sat together oohing and aahing and laughing, praising Allah and feeling altogether very good indeed. The mother and father and Yatsoua were bubbling with gratitude, enjoying the moment as much as we. We sent them off finally and came back into the house and shook hands on this little but lovely victory. "You probably didn't notice," Myra said (it is the phrase she uses when she is about to point out to me some colorful pattern on a woman's cloth, *or the unusual beads on someone's necklace, or the beautiful wildflowers in a field), "but he had the cutest little feet," and she curved her hand to show how they were. I hadn't, in fact, noticed, but I guess what she meant was she was glad he was alive, and it seemed as good a way as any of saying it.*

There Are Times When I Really Hate This Work

AT THE END of February, our Land Rover arrived. Gorgeous and strong, her diesel engine purred with profound determination, and she took our roads with little more difficulty than a motorboat on quiet waters. We bid an unfond farewell to the clouds of dust that had poured into our little Renault 12 and swirled chokingly and relentlessly around us. No more, we hoped, would a morning in the villages leave us with stiff white hair, powdered brown cloth, rattled teeth, and shattered nerves.

Our work, already progressing nicely, would sail even through the rainy season now. We were seldom anything less than exhausted at the end of the day, but it was a good exhaustion as gratifying successes with very sick children could make the most grueling, sweat-soaked day fun.

On the twenty-seventh of February President Bush announced a suspension of hostilities in Kuwait and Iraq. In Kolofata we had been alone in knowing and agonizing about what had been going on there, and we were alone in feeling the jubilation the day brought. But we felt we must be at one with the sentiments of Americans at home and abroad, rejoicing in the relief and praying that the end might truly mark the beginning of a new and better world.

Thursday, 14 March 1991

It has been six weeks now since I've had a letter, and I know it hasn't been six weeks since you last wrote. Everything coming to us is opened and sloppily resealed. That is better than not reaching at all but still grates on our American nerves.

We are working steadily through long hours in the dust and the heat and the gusting oven-hot winds. The people see fit to give us precious little rest—which is wonderful, of course, and why we are here, and I would have it no other way, but it is not easy. They wait for us on our front step in the morning when we get up, they stop us on the way to our village-of-the-day, they keep us going in bush through midday and then at the clinic until after dark and we are creeping around with flashlights, and invariably we no sooner get home at 7 or so than our verandah fills up with more women and sick kids. In between we have to somehow find time to cook, to boil and filter water, to clean and wash clothes, to balance the books and update the records and prepare the bottles and boxes for the next day. Oh, and to write letters. Did I forget sleep? We have given up dinner altogether. We grab a piece of fruit or some peanuts or a boiled egg and swallow them somewhere in between the evening's patients.

We spent a lovely morning today with M. Ali. This is his third visit to Kolofata since we've been here. He never spends more than a couple of days. And he is always inundated by people coming to him with problems. He has a native son's knowledge of and fondness for this area and the people. I have sensed that the many things he has done and sacrificed for them have gone largely unappreci-ated by the people—a man of wealth and stature can never do enough, but he is widely respected and recognized as a good man.

We have seen some grotesque malnutrition among the children. The treatment of malnutrition is complicated and multifaceted and at the moment we do not have the means and are not set up to deal with severe cases. The two year old girl carried to our house Wednesday night was so bloated her feet were like boiled sausages about to burst through their skins. Her eyelids, pussy and raw, were swollen shut. Her mouth was deeply cracked at the corners and her lips and gums and tongue were bright red with sores. Deep raw fissures marked every flexion crease on her body, and elsewhere her skin was peeling off in sheets, as if she were being flayed alive. In contrast to the swelling of her legs and face, her upper arms were scarcely bigger round than my thumb. She could not eat or drink, and the slightest movement of any part of her body caused her to scream in pain. Her grandmother held her there on our front step and asked me what to do.

There are times when I really hate this work. Or maybe it is not the work but the reality with which the work forces us to come into contact. A two year old girl who never did anyone any harm, who never brought anyone anything but smiles, dying a wretched, smelly, painful death because her parents were too poor or—more likely—too ignorant to prevent it. But the world is like that, isn't it. It's just that it doesn't have to be.

Saturday, 7 April 1991

A new recipe to tack into your files, particularly relished in time of famine:

Ingredients:

3 buckets dried cattle dung

½ bucket water

Materials:

clay pot with strainer holes punched in bottom

fire

Preparation time:

4 hours (including dung collection)

Method:

Place collected dung in a pile and set fire to it, burning to cinders.

Allow ash to cool slightly and spoon into clay strainer.

Take boiling water and pour over cinders.

Collect filtered drips in separate clay receptacle under strainer.

Mix this rich brown nourishing bouillon with your favorite leaves or roots and serve to friends and family on those special occasions . . .

I'm told it tastes a bit piquant and salty—a sort of beef broth with a difference—but I've not tried it. I've so far drawn the line at fried termites.

The other day having parked the vehicle in the sun all morning in one village (there were no trees) our two back tire tubes burst. We lost both at once, which was not fun. One spare serves two flats poorly.

We have had a horrendous week, flats aside. Started Easter morning when the chief from one of our villages came asking to have the vehicle sent out to pick up a woman from his village who had suddenly fallen seriously ill during the night. I sent Bello and he came back an hour later with two patients, a five year old girl whose temperature was through the roof and her thirty-fivish year old mother whose temperature was further through the roof and who was comatose and twitching besides. I will not relive the details—they exhaust me—but within the next 48 hours we had on our hands five cases of meningitis from two neighboring villages of Shuwas, one of the smaller tribes in the area who speak Arabic, and twenty or thirty people camped out on our compound. One man was just getting his IV put in [when] he gasped his last, and in the middle of a moonless night we drove the Land Rover packed with his corpse and crying chanting praying screeching relatives back to his village to be buried. The other four have done well, though the first woman is only now coming out of her delirium and starting to make sense. She has a 3 month old boy who is adorable. She has been a tough case, but I think she's going to be okay. The day after we realized that we had the start of an epidemic on our hands, we went out to the two villages and vaccinated. That was the day the tires burst.

For Muslims, Ramadan, the ninth month of the lunar year, is a time for fasting, prayer, and reflection. Ramadan traditions differ widely throughout the Muslim world, but in Kolofata day and night were essentially reversed. Two or three substantial meals were eaten during the night, and then nothing was ingested from the rising of the sun to its setting. The repudiation of daytime consumption was taken so literally that many people refused to swallow their saliva. Constant expectoration was the result.

Monday, 15 April 1991

The end of Ramadan at last today, and we are glad to see it over. The question is how long it will take people to break their monthlong habit of spitting, lying inert all day under the trees, and complaining of their terrible suffering. I see few toothpick limbs among our townsfolk after their month of alleged abstinence from food and drink, but I know that the doctor is fitting into a slim trim

90-pound package these days and Myra is back down to within 5 pounds of her slimmest-ever Naka self. But the point even if it were known would be lost on the people. Myra keeps saying she wants a t-shirt emblazoned with the words "I survived Ramadan."

The feast day today was quiet. AA normally comes back to Kolofata to celebrate with his people this most important of all Muslim holidays, but the troubles in Yaoundé prevented him from making it this year. Apparently he is the source of much of the feasting normally—he has countless cows, goats and chickens slaughtered for the people, and open house for all—and his absence put a damper on things and meant no feast for many.

The problems in Yaoundé threaten to be serious. The people have been making increasing demands for a multiparty system, and the president, though making progress toward such a system, is responding too slowly for large sectors of society. There have been demonstrations and violence, most of it down south. The so-called opposition is fragmented into more than a dozen would-be parties, making the obvious victor, should the current administration topple, the military. I am all for democracy and liberty and prosperity and everything else the rabble-rousers say they are for, but burning, looting and rioting seem an odd and inauspicious way of getting there, and they seem to forget how much more likely it is that massive sudden change will be for the worse than for the better.

We took in a woman for a few nights last week. Total body exhaustion. About 35, maybe 40. She had just delivered her 19th child, prematurely at 7 months, in bush. Twins, actually. Both had died within a day, and she came after the fact. She has one living child, a nine year old boy with sickle cell anaemia. Ten of her children had been twins. These were the first ones she delivered prematurely. All the others, twins and singletons, she had carried to term and they had died one by one at various ages, a week, nine months, three years . . . Eighteen sons and daughters, snip snip snip like flowers in a field. And the young sickler who remains will not live long. She was tired. Not just tired. Spent. As if all her life had flowed from her, down to these last two feeble drops, only to soak uselessly into the earth. The boy is good. But his eyes are yellow where they should be white and his tongue is bloodless and his head is the heavy bossed head of a sickler. He is not so well, she said to me as he crouched at her side. No, I said, but he is good, and I could think of nothing to add that made any sense.

This week we have been caring for a young—twentyish—Fulani shepherd who made the mistake of falling asleep while his goats and sheep wandered through the onion field of a Kanuri farmer. The farmer took his machete and whacked the young shepherd a dozen times over the head, then left him to die. Several hours later he was discovered, and several hours after that he was brought to us, comatose, limp and bleeding. Three limbs completely paralyzed, head the size of a carved pumpkin, assorted other gashes. Last night his heart slowed down a notch, and this morning one of his pupils is wide as the ocean, and the gaze of the two eyes is out of sync, and in spite of the fact that outwardly he looks the same—he lies there quietly, breathing peacefully, neither warm nor cool to the touch, and the flesh wounds are not so angry any more—in spite of all that, inside his skull he is dying. He is not going to make it. And it seems so silly. Here they cannot keep half their children alive because of all the natural hazards among which they live, and a young man who has made it through the prickly maze of childhood is clubbed to death for the sake of a few onions. It happens, they say, over and over again every year.

We are both well, enjoying excellent health in spite of—because of?—the constant drain on our time and energy. I am not sure that there is not some advantage conferred by quite simply not having the time to be sick.

The heat continues. 102° in our cool house yesterday. One's thirst is never quenched, and it is a struggle keeping up with the quantity of water that must be boiled and filtered to drink.

The Swift Ticking of a Little Heart

Sunday, 28 April 1991

Work is endless. (A bird just tapped at the door. Even the birds here tap at our door.) It is hard to see how we are going to bring the chaos under control. It must be two months since I have run with any regularity—for the first time in my life I cannot find that half hour chunk to cut out of my day. Finding time to eat and sleep is struggle enough—as frequently lost as won. We keep saying we are going to draw the line, limit the number of patients we can treat in a day, cut out a village or two, answer no more knocks at the door after a certain hour. But. They're sick. They hurt. Often they are or would be dying. Our choice is distressingly simple: either you stop caring or you do like you do round about mile 20, just keep putting one foot in front of the other and the other in front of that and wait and see if you drop.

We wondered if we would ever again be able to get enough sleep or rest or peace of mind, and if so, what earth-shattering event would have to transpire to permit it. Our good fortune was having too little time to think about it, and we were saved also by the delight we took in the people we served.

They lived as close to nature as one could live and knew things about plants and animals that a Westerner would have to study long and hard to learn. They tended to have a great deal of respect for machines. They enjoyed watching things like the needle of a sphygmomanometer bump down or the wheel on a scale whirl around to a stop. There were patients who seemed to feel instant relief when a stethoscope was placed over their chest. On occasion my obstetrical Doppler was helpful in dispelling surprising beliefs about pregnancy, as in cases of women who were convinced they had been pregnant for years.

On other occasions it helped in other ways. I was visiting a mission clinic in a neighboring district when a nurse asked me to see a forty-two-year-old woman who had never been pregnant but who now had missed her period for two months and was desperately hopeful to know if she was pregnant. The nurse thought that menopause was almost surely the explanation for her missed menses, and given her story of lifelong infertility, that seemed right to me. We had no rapid pregnancy tests in those days, but I told the nurse I would be happy to see this woman: maybe by putting the Doppler to her abdomen I could help her understand that menopause, not pregnancy, was upon her.

She was dressed in green and yellow cotton cloth, and her head and neck were veiled. She leaned forward in her straight-backed chair and looked unblinkingly at me as I talked to her. After confirming that she had never had children, no miscarriage, no pregnancy of any kind, she told me that although her periods were usually regular, two months had passed now with nothing.

"Do you think you are pregnant?" I asked.

"Well," she admitted, looking down for the first time, "I don't know. I have never been pregnant, and look at me, I am old. My time has passed." She paused to think. "But"—she looked up again—"yes, maybe. You will tell me."

I dreaded telling her what I would have to tell her.

She lay down, and I palpated her flat abdomen. I showed her the Doppler and tube of gel and explained to her how the machine worked. I told her the gel might be a little cold, but nothing would hurt, and then, bracing myself to give her the sad news that there was not, after all, a child inside, I put the earpieces in my ears, laid the instrument end on her belly, and pushed the button. Immediately the swift ticking of a little heart trickled into my head.

I felt the woman's pulse to be sure the beats did not coincide, and as they did not, I declared, "There is a baby in there!"

The woman, her lips trembling, suppressed a smile and wiped a traitorous tear from her eye. Forty-two was old age in our part of the world, and this woman had spent nearly thirty years of married life under the harsh stigma that is the lot of childless women in Africa. I prayed that God and all his angels might be in their heaven and paying very close attention over the next thirty weeks.

There Are No Bridges

Thursday, 16 May 1991

The seasons have changed. Preceding the first tentative rains, we [have] had incredible mid-afternoon dust storms. At two o'clock in the afternoon [Tuesday] it became dark as night, the wind raging, the air swirling with dense clouds of dust. Within minutes everything in our sealed house was coated with dirt. Roofs of huts and houses blew off, electric poles came crashing down, the temperature plummeted to eighty degrees—a swift drop of thirty or forty. Dust so thick you taste it when you breathe creeps through every pore and crack and crevice of whatever cover is supposed to be protecting instruments, needles, microscope, [and] a roomful of thirty sick men, women and children.

Once, out on the road, you could see the razor-sharp edge of the storm—on one side was sunlight, on the other darkness—as you approached it, gritting your teeth and gripping the wheel. The wind and the dust smacked against the vehicle as we entered, and visibility with headlights was about five feet.

Yesterday, after the fourth such storm, came the payoff: a luscious rain that lasted on and off for three hours. Heavy. We were in bush, at our farthest station. By the time we made our way back to Kolofata we were plowing through puddles the size of small lakes, creeping along at 10–15 MPH and nevertheless slipping and sliding as if the earth were ice. Not many vehicles would have made it at all, but the Land Rover kept chugging along and we got home without once getting stuck or punctured. Apart from washed-out bush "roads" there is a river (stream really but they call it a river) at the entrance/exit of Kolofata which floods and completely cuts us off for days at a time, and they say even the Land Rover will not be able to cross.

Following World War I, Cameroon, formerly a German colony, was divided between the victorious French and English. In 1955 the Union des Populations Camerounaises (UPC) incited widespread revolt, demanding independence. This was granted by both France and England with apparent glee, as neither country was ignorant of the drain their colonial charge had become on their economies. Supported by the French, Ahmadou Ahidjo, a northern Muslim, became president and ruled with little tolerance for dissent.

Ahidjo's protégé and prime minister, Paul Biya, a southern Christian, engineered a consensual transfer of power in 1982 and became president. Two years later Ahidjo, disappointed with Biya's comportment and egged on by his northern supporters, tried to stage a comeback, but the insurrection was put down. Ahidjo was sentenced to death, a thousand people lost their lives, and hundreds of others were thrown in prison where many would languish uncharged for six years.

Biya ruled with an ever more clenched iron fist in a one-party state until 1990, when the clamoring for democratic reform, spurred by local opposition and Western powers, became more and more strident. The stalling of a plan to legalize opposition parties led in 1991 to a campaign of civil disobedience. "Operation Ghost Town" called for the voluntary closure of all businesses, markets, and transportation services from Monday through Friday until the government gave in.

Sat, 18th May. More troubles in the country, this time striking in Mora—too close to home. Several buildings and vehicles burned, others smashed with sticks and rocks, numerous people injured and two killed when the gendarmes shot "warning shots" into the air. Lots of arrests, mostly teenagers. It seems that this has been the pattern in violence breaking out in cities throughout the country: opposition elements who have a vested interest in destabilization pay kids and down-and-outs to go around lighting fires and throwing rocks through windows. It works well, and I imagine it is a technique tried and true all over the world. The vast masses have no idea what is going on. They only see that all is not well. Or they see that a gendarme shot and killed a 17 year old boy. When AA was here last—he is chief of the gendarmes, like our National Guard, except in francophone countries a much more powerful, pervasive presence—he said that this was what gave him sleepless nights: the task of keeping his men from firing, particularly in the face of blatant provocation. And now a couple of kids have been killed next door in Mora. Matawa flew in yesterday, and with him came a team of 4 gendarmes from Maroua, rifles and all, to add a little muscle to the already hefty multiple-man guard that watches over the compound 24 hours a day. One of these guards now plants himself outside our front door at night.

The beefed up security has not deterred the sick from slipping through the gates and coming to the house at odd hours. Yesterday we got home from work at almost 8:00 and were greeted by rifle-bearing military types, which was disconcerting, but I thought, Oh well at least we'll have a quiet evening. Nobody is going to come through those gates with all that army-green around. Ha ha. We no sooner sat down and popped the top off a bottle of Fanta than the taps at the door started. And this morning was no different. The people from the bush have no time for political unrest, and anyway I don't suppose a rifle is any more menacing than a bad bout of dysentery or pneumonia.

A 20 year old woman [with a] bright but wild one year old boy came [at dusk]—no electricity, remember. [She had] fallen while carrying an urn of water from the well. The wild one on her back had started kicking and screaming and thrown her off balance. As she fell, the clay urn broke and her right hand landed squarely on the cut edge, and between her weight and the weight of the wild one the force was enough to rip a deep 4 cm gash down her ring finger and to sever the little finger clean through the bone just before the joint connecting it to the hand. She came, pushed several miles on the seat of a bicycle, wild one strapped on her back, holding her right hand in her left. The finger was still attached by palm-side tissues, and it [looked like] blood loss had not been excessive, so we decided to go ahead and see if we could get it hooked back up. She was stoic. While I was sputtering curses against the fading glow of a flashlight and our lack of sterile conditions and having to use a crummy artery forceps instead of a needle driver to hold my needle, she lay there quietly, occasionally grimacing but never uttering a peep, turning now and then to allow the wild one to suckle when the nearly useless husband got tired of holding him. We were well into a moonless night by the time the suturing was done and a plaster splint was fixed in place. Off she went, and every day she trekked back in, wild one on her back, for a week. The hand defied all probability, healing beautifully, and she has good movement in the little finger. With the physiotherapy forced upon it in keeping the wild one under control, that is likely to improve. The bill came to almost ten dollars, and although the husband was happy to pay, he did at one point ask if he could hand over the wild one instead. The young mother smiled through the side of her mouth, knowing that however crazy we might be, we weren't that crazy. (His name is Kadi and my guess is his IQ is somewhere near the boiling point, and he'll probably be a goat-herder when he grows up.)

Amadou Ali

Since the beginning of time, Kolofata boys were destined from birth to spend their lives tending sheep and goats and hoeing millet fields. Amadou Ali would have been no exception but for the fact that his father had had a dispute with the village chief. The colonial government of the day required each chief to supply a quota of boys to send away to school. Kolofata parents did not want their children to go away to school. They wanted them to stay in the village to tend the family's animals and hoe the family's fields. A savvy chief who wished to punish one of his subjects had the right to oblige the offender to surrender a son to be educated. The sentence was a harsh one dreaded by parents, and Ali's father, his protests failing to placate the chief, suffered this fate.

School was twenty-five miles away, and Ali (baptized Ali Amadou: a clerk later in life reversed his two names and Ali never changed it back; officially he became Amadou Ali, though family and friends continued to call him Ali) hated it. Whenever he saw a chance to escape, he took it, returning to Kolofata on foot. He was caught each time and brought to the village chief, who locked him up in a room in the palace and the next day sent him back to the city.

In spite of his many absences, Ali excelled in class and on exams and eventually discovered that excelling was something he enjoyed. He stopped trying to escape. He started accumulating honors. He stayed in school and completed his studies, including a stint at France's elite Ecole Nationale d'Administration. Back in Cameroon he entered the civil service and worked his way up the ranks through various ministries, becoming in turn head of the gendarmerie, minister of defense, presidential chief of staff, minister of justice, and finally, in 2004, vice prime minister.

He was good at numbers. Eschewing crutches like electronic contact lists on the grounds that they induced mental laziness, he kept scores of telephone numbers in his head. He knew the dates of hundreds of events in his life, in the lives of those around him, and in the life of his country. He remembered exact prices and the ins and outs of budgets going back decades.

Every few months he returned to Kolofata to reconnect with his roots and to try to help solve local problems. On occasions when his visit coincided with a holiday or celebration of some event, the town's dusty streets were clogged with cars, taxis, and buses bearing people who had come to see him, well-wishers and favor-seekers hailing from both sides of the border and hundreds of kilometers away. Closing his door to no one, he listened to the comments and pleas of each group, one after the other, and he sat up into the early hours of the morning, sometimes all night, to hear them out.

Ali was six feet two inches tall, and his stiff cylindrical bonnet added another four inches to his height. In later years he developed an administrative paunch, but as a young man and well into his sixties he was lean and athletic. The deep parallel lines carved into each cheek during infancy had darkened with age and lent him a dignity grounded in centuries of unbroken tradition. He wore neither mustache nor beard. In public he favored traditional dress of cotton pants and tunic covered by a massive *gondora*, or outer garment, elaborately embroidered and impeccably pressed. His shoes were pointed and polished. He moved with deliberate slowness at all times: walking fast was indecorous, fraught, a sign of weakness.

It was because of the efforts and influence of Ali that Kolofata would eventually boast a hospital, a bridge, three primary schools, and two secondary schools.

A devout Muslim, he shared his annual harvest with widows, orphans, the destitute, and the disabled. When the town's mosque needed repairs, he had them done. He preached tolerance. Christians and nonbelievers were part of his suite. He yearned for ever more learning for himself and for others, and he gave aid to students of any faith or tribe who proved themselves willing to advance by working hard. He tried to find jobs for Kolofata's unemployed youth, regardless of their allegiance.

He forged links, brought people together: a journalist and a doctor, a high school principle and an army general, an influential businessman and a mayor, a government minister and a farmer. He enjoyed the company of diplomats, university professors, engineers, scientists, writers, and entrepreneurs, and he gleaned what knowledge and experience he could from each one. Dinner at his table was never boring and never short.

When in spite of ample incentives, the population of Kolofata resisted sending their children to school because of their fear that school would draw them away from core Islamic values, he sought funding and built an Ecole Franco-Arabe whose teachers included volunteer Islamic scholars and whose curriculum incorporated Islamic studies into traditional public school academics. He hoped that if parents were assured that their sons and daughters would study the Quran while learning to read and write, they would soften their opposition to education. He further hoped that the school would be a way of introducing children to the classical, tolerant Islam that he embraced. Amadou Ali seemed to spy, well before it was visible to most, the black oil slick of extremism already oozing toward sub-Saharan Africa from beyond the horizon.

He believed in the potential of Cameroon, even of its most desolate corners. On a dare, he tried to grow dates in Kolofata—something that had never been done before—and he succeeded. He planted grapevines to see if they would grow, and he studied the art of viniculture. He learned how to prune and stake the vines and, when the time came, how to harvest their fat, purple fruit.

He encouraged parents to vaccinate their children. In the early 1990s during the opening ceremony of a mass meningitis vaccination campaign, just at the moment when the songs and the speeches were done and the vaccinating was about to begin, the population, terrified of what they were being asked to submit to, turned tail and ran off in all directions. As he watched them scatter, Ali grabbed the microphone and called out to the crowd to wait, wait, come back, he had something to say. Recognizing his voice, men, women, and children stopped in their tracks, turned around, and inched back. Ali reminded them that he was one of them, a Kolofatan, a Kanuri, and how could they think he could bring anything to the village that would do them harm? He explained what had already been explained to them by the suits and ties from the capital—the goal of vaccination, the horror of meningitis—but this time in words the people understood, and then he rolled up his sleeve and asked the nurse to vaccinate him now, in front of everyone. This was done, and the crowd was won over. They came forward, jostling to be injected, and by the end of the day some had waited in two or three different lines and been vaccinated two or three times, figuring that if Ali said one shot was good, three must be very good indeed.

From time to time, particularly during his tenures as minister of defense and minister of justice, he received death threats. He said that he was not afraid of dying and was ready to go whenever his time came, but he did not want to die before that time; he did not want to die stupidly. He went yearly for medical checkups and kept his vaccinations up-to-date. He accepted, with reluctance but understanding, the security details assigned to him, though he chafed when even in Kolofata he could go nowhere unattended. "This is my hometown," he said. "Who would attack me here?"

Slipping and Sliding through the Mud

Sunday, 16 June 1991

AA came up this weekend primarily for a meeting in Maroua but secondarily to inaugurate [the] new "sports complex" he has nearly finished building at one end of his large compound. It is quite impressive, on a bush African scale. At one end is a stable designed to hold 4 horses. At the other end is a locker room. In the middle is a large cement court, painted red and green and lined in different colors to mark out courts for tennis, basketball, volleyball and European handball. He has assorted dignitaries and 6 volleyball teams in from Mora and Maroua today for a tournament. Before it started he was out there with a few other adults and a dozen urchins from the village having a grand time playing a pickup game of volleyball. It was lovely to see. He is really a village boy at heart, for all his pomp and grandeur. I think that if at any moment you gave him the choice of being out on that court with that band of ragamuffin boys or sitting regally gowned and bound in the back of a chauffeur-driven black Mercedes he would not hesitate to choose the former. The tennis court should be ready in a few weeks.

The clinic is in pretty good condition, although we were flooded out with the early heavy rains. After a struggle we got the roof repaired but it still is not waterproof and needs more work. I want to put up a new building as a first step toward developing a real hospital. Housing patients on our doorstep gets the job done, in a fashion, but it is not ideal.

The young Cameroonian doctor left long ago. The nurses cannot be trusted to give medicines as ordered, to show up to work sober, or to show up to work at all. All are outsiders who do not speak the local languages and are inordinately proud of the fact. The stories I could tell you . . . The people in general hate the [old hospital] and will not go. Yet they come in droves to us up the hill, and the majority are people who have never been to see a doctor or a nurse. The confidence they show in coming, therefore, is not a small thing, and it must be carefully nurtured. This we feel we can only do by keeping our program out from under the dark shadows cast by the old. We are starting fresh, and if I had my druthers, the old would be obliterated, the nurses dismissed, the building converted to storage rooms and guest rooms for families of out-of-town patients. We would train a new team of local people whose interests are sincere and who would be held accountable for their actions—or inactions. It is crystal clear in my mind how such a program could develop, and we are taking early tentative steps. Politics [is] everywhere, though, and it is not easy to avoid stepping on toes.

Monday, 24 June 1991

Half an hour here before we have to go up. Yesterday was the Fête de Mouton—the "sheep holiday"—which is the celebration of Abraham's sparing his son. Everyone eats sheep. The whole point of the holiday is to eat to repletion and beyond. Fortunately, here among our Muslims, there is a minimum of alcohol going down at the same time. But we had bellyaches to treat in the middle of the night.

About ten days ago we were knocked out of our beds around midnight by the usual blasting at the door. Doors are foreign things and people seldom just tap and settle back to await a response. No. They POUND, first of all, and if there is no response within three nanoseconds, they POUND again. And then again. And again. Evermore vigorously, ever more impatiently, ever more demandingly. I fear for our door sometimes—and for my heart. It is no treat to be roused from a deep three-quarters dead sleep at midnight in this manner. The only way of getting the pounding to stop is to go open the door, but there is the minor detail of slipping on a frock first. I did eventually accomplish this little task—and the subsequent ones of groping for a flashlight (knocking it over and crawling to retrieve it after it had rolled under the bed—this is how it happens every time) and fumbling for the right key and getting it right side up into the keyhole—have you ever noticed how much smaller keyholes are at midnight than at noon?— and, ah yes, opening the door. Usually I open the door (remembering at the last minute to smooth down that pillow-peaked wave of hair on the top of my head) and am confronted by three or four persons who stand back in numbed silence (the malignant pounder is never self-evident) staring dumbly at me as if to say, "Oui, Madame, did you call?"

This night they were not shy. A man had been shot through the hand, very bad they said, and was there anything I could do. Of the four men there I saw none in great distress so I asked where he was. Lying out by the gate. I suggested they bring him in, and they did, a big strong giant of a man holding a wrapped hand dripping huge drops of blood and crying and whimpering like an injured puppy. His hand was a mess. It had been ripped apart at the heel and much of the palm had been blown off, skin, fat, muscle and all. Limp severed vessels gave forth steady streams of bright red blood; in short order the verandah was puddled with it. We got a table draped with plastic and set up under a light in our hangar and went to work. Apart from being an anatomical nightmare, the wound was full of grit and we spent our first hour or two just trying to clean it. And then we proceeded to make a sizable dent in our stock of sutures. Amazingly, the bones and joints were all intact, as was the essence of the hand's blood supply, and fortunately [his] was the thick meaty hand of a farmer. It was like trying to fit a fleshy jigsaw puzzle together [but with] an unknown number of pieces missing from the middle. I did what I could, saving as much skin as looked salvageable and trying to get the other tissues hooked up more or less like they were supposed to be. In the end a gaping crater was left in the middle, and it was not pretty, but we wrapped him up and gave him a couple of injections and an hour or so before dawn sent him off. Ten days later the stitches are out and the hand is still there, fairly normal looking and reasonably functional—except for that big crater which will be slow to heal. But with time it will.

As the rains picked up, we started having a few adventures trying to get to our villages. One Thursday morning in mid-July, with Bello at the wheel of the Land Rover, we hit a soft spot that had been hidden by grass and promptly sank. The Land Rover was a high vehicle with big tires, but the mud was dismissive of that. In an attempt to regain some forward motion, Bello nudged the accelerator, but his success was limited to spinning the wheels and burying half the chassis in the muck. Fortunately, he was a chipper worker and unlike me not easily upset by such trivial inconveniences as a Land Rover in the middle of nowhere under a hot midmorning sun sunk to its gills in mud and sinking inches deeper with every rescue attempt. We spent the next several hours trudging barefoot, occasionally tipping into knee-deep mud, swatting bugs, and trying to avoid trampling frogs, snakes, and scorpions as we scoured the paddy-like fields for bits of wood.

We wedged branches and chains under the tires and pushed and pushed and failed and failed and then started all over again. Two women passed by on their way to farm. They stopped to join our meager team, and they were kind and eager to help, but they were a little less than the force we needed. At last the posse came: ten men on bicycles from a village several miles away on the border with Nigeria. Though headed for a naming ceremony in Kolofata and dressed in pristine robes, they didn't hesitate. They laid their bicycles aside, took off their shoes and outer garments, rolled up their sleeves, and set to work. After reinforcing the traction, each one grabbed a piece of the vehicle and grunted and shoved and slipped and silently withstood the torrent of water and mud being thrown at them as Bello spun the wheels.

Finally, with one mighty heave, the monster moved up and out of the deep rut it was in—and smack into a new one. This time, however, one side was much deeper than the other so that a nearly forty-five-degree angle was struck, and it seemed all Bello had to do was breathe wrong for the passenger side to plop over onto the ground. The men appeared surprised by this development, but they were undeterred. They gathered on the tilted passenger side to keep it from going down and just continued pushing and shoving and ignoring the shower of mud that kept flying in their faces. By the time the Land Rover was freed from its mired crypt, they were drenched in mud from head to toe, as were we all. The men nonchalantly set about washing themselves and their clothes in puddles and then prepared to leave. I offered a token of gratitude—for their *goro*, or *kola*, I said, as was the custom—but they adamantly refused. "We didn't do it for you," they said. "We did it for us."

We continued on and reached our village, though too late to do any work. Instead we piled the worst cases in the Land Rover and carried them back to Kolofata with us—but this time by a different route.

The country was continuing to do its own slipping and sliding through the mud as calls for multiparty democracy became more and more strident. The bigger towns and cities were racked by strikes and riots. Buildings and cars were being burned. People were being shot and sometimes killed. The government responded by outlawing a number of organizations, including the main human rights organization, and jailing journalists and opposition leaders for allegedly inciting crowds to violence. The BBC reported that in the important market town of Maiganga, people were shooting poisoned arrows at one another in an outbreak of tribal warfare. As part of an effort to interrupt economic activity, the strategy of ghost towns, or *villes mortes*, succeeded for a while in shutting down many of the bigger cities, including Garoua and Maroua in the country's north. Protesters set fire to tires in the middle of the streets to keep people off the roads and out of shops, markets, and offices. Any place of business that dared to stay open got burned closed. Truckloads of uniformed men descended on the cities.

There were two things I found strange in all this, apart from the fact that it was happening at all. One was that these events were receiving almost no coverage by the Cameroon media. The other was that administratively, governmentally, life was going on as usual. Not only was there no attempt to appease protesters' demands, but the very existence of their demands was blithely ignored. Officials did not miss a beat in rolling out their usual ceremonies, campaigns, meetings, and seminars, giving not the slightest nod of recognition to the climate of unrest. Public health programs were pushed with vociferous enthusiasm. Routine agricultural agendas and interventions were promoted anew. In an apparent effort to leave civil servants with no time for their attention to stray, ever more voluminous reports of questionable value were demanded at every level. The band played on. If winds of change were in the air, the government seemed to be trying hard to be sure everyone understood they were no more than gentle breezes that would soon fade away.

As much as the rains were loved for the hope they gave our farmers, they were hated for the added hardships they brought. Mosquitoes swarmed. Electricity poles toppled. Walls crumbled. Roofs flew off. Fields flooded, destroying crops. When roads and paths washed out, people were locked in their villages for days at a time, and this at a particularly sick time of year when malaria, diarrhea diseases, and malnutrition were at their worst.

By August, the previously parched earth had sucked in all the moisture it could, so new rain accumulated and formed unbreachable lagoons. Once-solid ground turned to deep mud. The main causeway connecting Kolofata with the rest of the country flooded every time a hard rain fell, and the river, dry most of the year, ran high and flowed with a force that defied any attempt to cross. Water that swept around the crossing carved new paths in the sand, cutting to depths that could bury a man.

Chad-bound tankers laden with Nigerian oil had to pass through Kolofata, and their cocky drivers commonly misjudged their ability to overcome the current that roared over our causeway. They tipped midstream. Days would pass as efforts were made to pull a tanker out of the water, and it seemed that one tanker no sooner would be removed than another would come along and tip in its turn. Then even if the rains let up for a few days and the current subsided, no one could get through because of the work being done to remove the downed vehicles. As a consequence, a line of tankers waiting to get through town stretched for miles and stayed for days. Their drivers installed themselves on mats under their tanks and passed the time with cigarettes, *femmes libres* (prostitutes), and sleep.

When the current waned and the water descended enough to permit the heartiest to traverse the causeway, muscular young men skilled in the vagaries of the river made a decent daily wage by hefting people and goods onto their backs and lumbering across. Motorcycles as well were carried across this way, held high and dry on the shoulders and heads of valiant youths.

When in Doubt, Do Nothing, Go Nowhere, Say Not a Word

17 August 1991

A local woman at term with her fourth child (two living) started bleeding on Saturday and came to see me. The river was down, and I told her that [the need for] an operative delivery was a strong possibility [and I advised her to go to] Mora. She was reluctant, I thought, but said she would go home and tell her husband. I told her I was going to Mora the next day and if her bleeding didn't increase before then and she couldn't get transport she could come with us. Sunday [and then again] Monday [there was] no word [from her] until 5 PM when in a great panic four men carried her to the clinic and deposited her on my floor. She was pouring out blood and was shocky. They said she had started bleeding heavily in the morning and [they] gave no explanation of why nothing had been done either then or in the two days preceding. Inertia. It is a ghastly thing here. When in doubt, do nothing, go nowhere, say not a word. It cuts across all sectors of our closed little society. It had rained the night before, the river was up, and no vehicles were able to pass. We started a drip and got a stretcher and a vehicle and carried her down to the river. Four men carried her over the river, drip and all, and another vehicle took her from the other side to the next river where they had to cut the engine and have the truck pushed across. Her good fortune could only have been miraculous, for she made it to Mora and they operated and saved her life. The child—who had still been alive in Kolofata—was lost.

Bello, our driver, was sick all week so I was at the wheel getting to some of our most remote stations, four-wheel-driving through swamps and over flooded causeways. We got truly stuck only once and were sloshing barefoot through the fetid stagnant water to collect sticks and barehandedly digging mud out from under the sunken wheels, certain our tender ankles were being invaded by all manner of cercariae and other living creatures. Myra keeps saying that sometimes it is no fun being an MPH, knowing the biological dangers that lurk all around us to which she would otherwise be contentedly oblivious.

The American ambassador, Frances Cook, sent a care package up with AA for us. A big box stuffed with America's best M&Ms, crackers, granola bars, muffin mix, jams, perfume and powders and soaps, canned corn and sauerkraut. We were touched. Also a nice letter and information about a small fund available for community self-help projects and an invitation to think something up and get the community to apply—which we have started to do.

Tuesday, 27 August 1991

We used our obstetrical vacuum for the first time yesterday. A vacuum [is] what most people in the world use in cases when Americans use forceps. Like forceps it looks like something out of a medieval torture chamber. Never before has Kolofata seen such a thing. I was called down from a busy clinic to assess this woman who had been in long labor with her first child and who the nurses feared would have to go to Mora for a C-section. Nurses and assorted relatives [stood] around anxiously. The river up, no one [knew] if the road was passable beyond Kolofata. I examined her and said it looked like she ought to be able to push [the baby] out with coaching and maybe a bit of help. Our nurses have a habit of laughing at patients who find themselves in such difficulties, and one of them was doing so now, so I got our undynamic but sincere Abaram [one of our locally trained semiliterate health promoters] to coach and Myra to flex her muscles with the pump, and I fitted the business end on the baby's head and got up on a cement block because I was too short for the table, and like a finely tuned quartet we coached and pumped and pushed and pulled—and out eased a pink wriggling baby girl, hallelujah. Well done, well done, well done etc. to the mother. I asked the nurses if they could finish up, and yes they could, and the three of us hurriedly left to go back to our busy clinic. We were all pretty pleased.

He Was Burned Everywhere

Saturday, 31 August 1991

Darkness falls here around 6:30 these days. After a crowded and hectic morning and afternoon yesterday, we finished at the clinic at 6:45, loaded the Land Rover and headed toward the hospital to be sure all was quiet before going home. (A routine and necessary stop but also something of a joke, [for] rarely are any of the nurses supposedly on duty anywhere to be found.) The clinic is located on the west end of the village, the "hospital" on the east end, near the river. As we approached, a massive gust of black smoke went up somewhere in the vicinity of the river, and within seconds billowing orange flames filled the sky. They surged, so dense and expansive they looked like something solid, but too violent to be contained within a shape, like an artist's depiction of a close-up of the sun. Black smoke, the smell of gasoline, and then the screams of human beings.

People fled. Wild-eyed and looking over their shoulders. Men hopped on bicycles and pedaled, women grabbed what children they could find and ran. We heard snatches: a tanker loaded with gasoline overturned at the river, and it and dozens of drums full of fuel all around it were blowing up. The river is a place where children play all day, and parents who could not find their sons and daughters were panic-stricken. The rest were just scared and running, hundreds and hundreds of them, already resigned to the fate of their village which was about to be devastated. They ran for miles. Everyone told us to get [our] vehicle out of town. The fire lit the smoky horizon, and every time it seemed to settle a little a new explosion regurgitated fresh flames.

And then came news of the first casualty, a six year old boy. We went to the house to load up drips and gauze and needles, and then back to the clinic. They carried him in wrapped in a cloth—his own clothes had been burned off him.

Already he was icy cold. He was burned everywhere. Everywhere. Head to toe. Face, ears, scalp, all four limbs, his torso front and back. Charred skin hung in long sheets off his little body. His whole face was flayed and red. I doubt that more than 10% of his body surface was spared. Yet he was lucid, talking in his little boy voice through lips that were bubbling and swelling before our eyes. He did not complain of pain. He was thirsty and wanted water please. He said he had been by the drum of gasoline and he kept falling down, and could he have some water please. I could find no veins in his hands or his feet but his femoral vein at the groin gave access and we started pouring fluids into him, and we shut the windows and piled sheets and towels on him in the room which must have been near 100° F. We trimmed off the larger sheets of burned skin and when he got very restless and uncomfortable we gave him an intravenous painkiller. We stayed with him and talked to him and tried to understand the garbled words that came through his swollen mouth, and we gave him little sips of water, first through a blue cup then through a syringe, then through the cup again when he said really he would prefer to have his water from the blue cup.

His father—a non-Kolofatan, a civil servant from down south working in the customs office here—was there, and an older brother, and various other people wandered continuously in and out. The father kept telling him not to worry, he was going to get better. He also grilled the boy several times, asking whether anyone had pushed him or made him fall—vengeance clearly foremost in his mind. The boy insisted over and over that no one had pushed him, he was by the drum and he just kept falling, and could he have some water please.

He did not have a chance. After four hours he gently slipped into coma and moments later he died.

I'd had visions of our town being razed to cinders in the night, perhaps within hours, but the holocaust never happened. The tanker had fallen in such a way that it was surrounded by water—deep wide gullies where the heavy rains had cut new channels, transecting the road in several places. That water, and surely the grace of God, saved us. The fire burned all night, but it never leapt that island of rock on which the tanker lay. Injuries, too, were mostly minor, with the exception of our boy and one five year old girl who while running away was struck by a motorcycle and had half her right cheek ripped off. She came in while we were working on the boy and in the darkness I patched her up as best I could, matching the pieces of jigsaw. On an ordinary day it would have been a horrible thing to see, but with the boy lying beside her skinless, his life oozing out of him, it seemed little more than an abrasion.

Two of our new local health workers showed up and were a big help. Three nurses who were not on duty did likewise—the first time I have seen any spark of initiative from them. On the other hand, the nurse who was supposed to be on duty we passed outside her home as we were going up to the clinic. She had rescued her refrigerator and a small carton of something and was standing there, presumably waiting to be carried off with her possessions by a gallant knight. We saw no more of her that night or the next day. (Being Sunday now.)

When the work was over and the mess somewhat cleaned up, we came home to sleep. I could not close my eyes without images lighting up like flares—mushroom clouds of flame and smoke, fleeing hordes, peeling skin, the swollen body, lipless mouth, and always the smell of gasoline and leaking plasma and burned flesh.

Saturday morning the sun rose and the sky was clear and only the charred skeleton of the tanker burned quietly, unspectacularly, on, four or five isolated, ridiculously impotent-looking flames. Villagers went about their morning activities gaily, fetching water, washing clothes, setting out their little piles of beans and leaves and limes to be sold. Children ran and played, everyone shouted greetings. Sons and daughters had all been accounted for—some had fled as far as neighboring villages several miles away—and property had been unscathed. Even the millet in the fields bordering the river still stood. Everything about the morning was normal—or maybe a little better than normal. But the normalcy itself was eerie, the child dead and the near utter devastation of the night before so quickly and easily set aside.

Tuesday, 10 Sep. I had fried grasshoppers for breakfast yesterday. Seems to be the season. I was happy enough with my bread and jam today.

Life is so fragile. Stay close to one another. I love you very much.

E

There Is Sure to be Sorcery Involved

Amadou Ali's father, the father's three wives, and some of their children and grandchildren lived in the compound next to ours. In addition to the family homes, extra rooms and huts were always filled with people passing through—distant relatives, old friends, acquaintances of acquaintances—who sometimes stayed for years.

Hadja Mairam was Ali's mother and the father's first wife. She was as tiny and self-contained as her husband and famous son were towering and expansive. Devoutly religious, she was respected by Kolofatans for her age and wisdom, her spiritual demeanor, and her wealth of knowledge about indigenous ways of treating illness.

Gana was a ten-year-old boy who had been informally adopted by Hadja Mairam when his mother abandoned him after the death of his father. Ali maintained that he thought his mother was crazy to do this, but my impression was that deep down he respected her for it, as he respected her for the hospitality she offered many people, related or not, who for whatever reason were in need of shelter and food for a while.

Gana had a cherubic smile and lively demeanor that endeared him to us. When not in school, he came to bush with us and often helped with odd jobs around the compound or clinic. He fried us our first grasshoppers. He performed in the educational skits our promoters staged in the clinic's waiting room. He had a habit of asking wonderful questions. Once he caught a pair of birds, and when they were taking too long to reproduce, he asked Myra if she could give him some medicine that might get them going.

One morning as we were at home and about to leave for the clinic, I came out of my room and found Myra sitting on the couch, looking bemused.

"We seem to have a cultural problem on our hands," she said, and then went on to explain that Gana had just come to the door requesting some of her or my hair so that Hadja Mairam could cure a sick child. He had insisted that we didn't have to cut it; it could just come off a comb or a brush.

This sounded strange, but not uninteresting. I went to the door, called Gana over, and asked him what the problem was.

"It is the problem," he said, "of the hair."

I asked him what that meant, and he repeated his story, that Hadja Mairam had sent him to get some hair from one of us because there was a child whose heart was beating. Beating of the heart was a common complaint that generally meant a person's heart was pounding so hard or so fast—as from fever, for example, or anemia—that the pulsations were unusually felt or visible at the chest wall.

Gana added that the normal cure of putting charcoal on the child's chest had not worked, so Hadja Mairam was going to try a different cure using our hair.

We were new to Kolofata, and although we were learning quickly, we were a long way from understanding all the cultural nuances that might help us determine what we should or should not do in a situation like this. On the one hand we did not want to cross or even question an elder as widely respected and influential as Hadja Mairam. On the other hand, the request seemed bizarre. In the end, we could not think of a reason to refuse, so I told Gana that we could give him a few strands of hair on condition that he tell Hadja Mairam that if the child was very sick or if the hair cure did not work, she send him to me, so I could see if he needed other treatment as well. Gana agreed, and Myra lifted some filaments off her brush, wrapped them in a swatch of paper, and gave the packet to him. Off he went.

This was in the morning, and neither of us thought more about it until late in the day when Bello came up and asked Myra what Gana had been doing at our house that morning. She recounted the story, and Bello, fuming, declared that Gana had lied and that somebody in town had paid him to do what he did.

"There is sure to be sorcery involved," he stated. He was furious, and so were our health workers. They stormed down into the village, got Gana to identify the man who had sent him on his quest, and yanked the culprit up to the clinic to explain himself.

His name was Cherif, and he looked about eighteen years old. He was a Kolofatan preparing to return to Maroua to finish his last year of high school. This made him highly educated by local standards and already a member of the town's "elite." Cherif flatly denied everything, but news of what was evidently going to be a scandal spread instantly. The consensus was that someone was trying to practice witchcraft on the white doctors. Cherif was hounded through the night so relentlessly that by morning he had no choice but to admit his guilt. He explained that he had told Gana to go to our house, tell the story about Hadja Mairam and the sick child, and come back with our hair. Cherif added that he too was only acting on the orders of someone else, but he refused to say who that person was. The townspeople were convinced it was a marabout, and the prevailing thought was that Cherif had gone to the marabout for help getting into the police academy, which everyone knew he dearly wanted, and the marabout had planned to devise a charm or a spell that involved some body part—hair would do—from one of the two white medics.

With people believing that Myra and I were the targets of evil intent, the matter was not allowed to rest. The *sous-préfet* was informed and ordered the local gendarmerie commandant to open an inquiry and arrest whoever needed to be arrested. The mayor of Mora was informed and sent investigators of his own. Amadou Ali, in France on state affairs, was called and ordered other gendarmes to Kolofata to investigate and take action as needed.

The gendarmes wanted us to register a formal complaint, alleging attempted witchcraft. We declined repeatedly, despite the intervention of the *sous-préfet*, who urged us to file so that an official investigation could be opened and the culprits brought to justice. Sorcery, he explained, was a crime punishable by six years' imprisonment.

"In addition," he insisted, "if anything happens to you, we will be called before the embassy of the United States and asked to explain why we did nothing to save you when we knew this thing was happening."

Myra and I were less afraid of being spelled upon than perhaps we should have been, and so we still declined to file suit.

"All it would take," the *sous-préfet* confided, "is a few lashes on this boy's back and he will talk."

This disinclined us even more to complain.

Three burly gendarmes from Mora showed up the next night and, over beers and cigarettes, sat down with us in the front room of one of Amadou Ali's small guesthouses. Windows and doors were closed to discourage eavesdroppers. Whorls of smoke and whiffs of Guinness filled the air. The job of recording what everyone else said fell to a gendarme whose longhand script seeped with the speed of molasses from pen to paper. In order not to outpace him, every question and answer had to be given one word at a time. The officers spent more time bickering with one another over the wording of a question, the need for a question, or the justness of its grammar than they spent either asking or listening. When the note taker made a mistake, he crossed it out. When he forgot to record something, he added it in with the help of elaborate arrows and curlicued brackets. Sometimes he scrapped whole paragraphs and started them over again.

Every so often he asked me to read what he had written to be sure he had gotten it right. "My penmanship is quite good—better than a doctor's, don't you think?"

I did not tell him that his handwriting was deplorable, but it was.

Although we persisted in refusing to file a complaint, the authorities deemed that the practice of witchcraft presented enough of a threat to public security that they should pursue the matter to its end. The investigation involved much of the town giving witness to one thing or another, and in the end the marabout was identified and arrested. Gana's perfidy cost him his foster family, as Hadja Mairam expelled him from her home and sent him back to his village to fend for himself. Myra and I remained alive and well. Cherif, the instigator who had sought the marabout's help in the first place, succeeded in his final year of school, entered the police academy, and went on to enjoy a successful and profitable career as an officer of the law.

Of Donkeys, Sheep, and Stables

Sunday, 3 November 1991

This week was a tough one, with lots of patients and some very bad cases, and in the middle of it we put in an all-nighter trying to save a baby who died anyway at dawn, and at the end of it a mob-scene vaccination session at the clinic during which we nearly got trampled. In the old days, the word vaccination caused a stampede in the opposite direction. There has been time for nothing but plodding on, and we are back to our old problem of struggling to get enough to eat due to the lack of time and energy to do any cooking. We are subsisting on bread, cheese, olives and raw tomatoes. And coffee. Thank goodness for Cameroonian coffee.

Our political problems wax and wane. Douala and other parts of the country down there are in turmoil, but on the whole government and life continue as if nothing is going to change in any great hurry. AA says people finally looked around at the alternatives and realized they didn't want any of them for the time being. He may have a slightly over-optimistic view of things, but I think he is right in believing that any radical change is almost certain to make things worse.

In late November or early December, the harmattan winds started to blow down from the Sahara. Relative humidity dropped to 10 percent, and dust filled the air like smog. With the dust came the cold. Daytime temperatures still reached the eighties and nineties, but it seldom felt that warm, as the dust and the bleak white sky seemed to rob the sun of its heat. Then a chill settled over the nights. To fight it, people filled shallow clay bowls with burning coal embers and incense and brought them into the hut or the hospital room with them. In the mornings roadsides were lined with huddles of children crouched around tiny flames set to fistfuls of straw. Everyone piled on layers of cloths and scarves, and a necessary part of any morning greeting was "How is the cold?" to which the correct reply was "It is there."

Viruses and bacteria seeking fragilized respiratory tracts had a field day.

On a Wednesday morning in late November, two teenaged boys led a donkey to the hospital and tied it to a tree. They wore loose robes and molded plastic shoes, and each carried a long stick. Slung over the donkey's back was a third boy, about seven years old. The teens lifted the youngest off the donkey and carried him inside, where a nurse guided them straight to my consulting room. The older boys set the sick child on the examining table and then stood erect and anxious by his side.

The three were brothers, and the sick one's name was Abba. Their father had died some years earlier. Abba's neck arched so far rearward that the back of his head nestled between his shoulder blades and could not be nudged a centimeter forward. His skin was fiery hot, his breathing rapid and labored. He was skinny enough that the whole of his skeleton could be traced, and bed sores had worn through the skin at both hips.

After asking them a few questions and examining the patient, I explained to the older boys that their brother had meningitis and pneumonia and was in a very bad way, but I thought we could help him. I wrote up orders and called a health worker to carry Abba to the ward while the brothers went to the hospital pharmacy to collect the drips and medicines needed to start his treatment.

I continued seeing other patients and by chance happened to look out my window half an hour later. In the courtyard I saw the oldest brother untying the donkey from its tether and leading it to the door of the ward. He entered and seconds later came out again, carrying his ailing brother in his arms. I leaped out of my chair and rushed outside.

"What are you doing?" I asked him.

"We are going home," he replied, eyes downcast.

The bill for treatment had come to the equivalent of nearly twelve dollars, and this for them was out of reach. "We will sell our millet at market on Saturday, and if we get enough, we will bring Abba back."

I endeavored to make him understand that Abba would not make it to Saturday if they left now, and I asked him if they could leave something in hock, pay the cash later. As I said this, I eyed the gray beast of burden and hoped he would not suggest leaving that. He thought for a while and then gave a nod to the second brother, who disappeared around the other side of the building. Less than a minute later he came back, trailing a seatless, rimless bicycle.

"That will do fine," I said, and it did, and Abba, after a week of touch-and-go, did as well. On the day before discharge, the brothers came with a pocketful of coins. They were not enough to cover the bill, but they sufficed. The next day the middle brother pedaled while the others perched atop the faithful donkey. Side by side, the three of them set off down our hill. I marveled at how easily and for how little this perfectly fine boy could have been lost.

Donkeys always made me think of Christmas, and every Christmas I enjoyed believing there was one patient sent to us specially for the season. That second Christmas in Kolofata our baby Jesus was a month-old girl who was the only living child of a woman who had already buried seven sons and daughters. Suffering severe malnutrition, the girl weighed four and a half pounds. Some of that paltry weight was no more than retained water ballooning her feet and filling the small of her back with a sickening bogginess. She had flaking skin and dull, rolling eyes.

Her mother claimed she did not have enough breastmilk, but it did not take us long to realize that what she really meant was that she had been giving her child no milk at all. This was a common conundrum. Mothers who had lost young children were often told by marabouts and elders that their milk was bad and that bad milk was the cause of their children's deaths. Such mothers were advised to withhold breastmilk from any subsequent progeny, and so convinced were they of the soundness of this counsel that changing their minds was always an arduous, frustrating, and time-consuming process. Mothers had to be persuaded not only that their milk was not bad but that withholding it would likely be lethal. They had to accept that the marabouts and old sages were wrong. Then if in the end they expressed willingness to believe but their child died anyway, they had to risk being blamed for yet another death.

The woman was in rags, the child had no clothes at all, and the hospital was still not much more than a stable. We took them in, bought the baby a tin of infant formula, and nursed her back to health. She responded brilliantly, and by Christmas she had gained enough weight that in the right light we were sure we could see a dimple begin to wink in her cheek. All the while we cajoled the mother, urging her to put the child to her breast, for none of us had enough money to keep buying formula for long. The mother resisted, trying as hard to make us understand her concern as we were trying to make her understand ours. Then, tentatively and fearfully, she gave in. Once she put her daughter to her breast, it did not take long for the milk to return. Her baby latched onto it like a drowning man to a ladder, and we watched her grow and glow with new life. By the time they left to go back to their village, no sign of deprivation remained. Her grateful mother seemed to have shed all doubt, and we just hoped she was staunch enough to face the critics who surely awaited her at home.

Friday, 3 Jan 92. And so out with the old. Happy New Year. I know you have suffering of your own, what with snow and ice and so on, and truly you have all my sympathy and you cannot possibly have any for me—but it is bloody cold here these days. My nose feels like an icicle, my toes are numb, my fingers are stiff, my blasted pen won't write. 59 degrees this morning, kid you not. I down hot coffee and all I get for it is a full bladder rendered all the more impatient by the chill in the air. The harmattan blew in with a fury two days ago, and it is fierce. Fine fine dust is everywhere. It creeps through the threads of your clothes and fills the creases in your skin. Visibility is no more than a couple hundred meters—if you strain the eyes. The sun, defeated, is only a vague glow more or less located in one spot in the pale white sky. The wind whips. Three, four times a day you dust, and still each time you lift a book its imprint is there again, outlined in white powder. Patients keep pans of burning charcoal by their bed. We delivered a prem baby the other day and wrapped him in a mountain of towels and cloths and blankets. I think we all secretly envied him. Anyway I did. Respiratory tract infections soared in December. The landscape all around is barren, colored only in shades of beige and undappled by shadows.

A boy, seventeenish, from Kolofata, speaks French, goes to school, came yesterday to see me. Neck puffed out like a bullfrog's, so much that he could only open his jaws a crack. Feverish, faint. I got a tongue depressor between his teeth and pried enough to get a light to shine in. The back of his throat was beet-red and dripping with pus and swollen nearly shut. Seems he'd had a sore throat on Sunday and was advised by his brother to go to the barber to have his uvula cut out. So this he did. Only much to his surprise and chagrin, instead of going away, the sore throat got worse.

People here don't, in general, like uvulas. They think they make babies vomit and grow thin, so they [take] their infants to the barber to have their throats slit. Sometimes I mention that it probably isn't a great idea, and they nod politely and say things like "oh ho" and then go out and do it anyway. For the moment we have to be content that they then come to us to pick up the pieces.

Thursday, 16 January 1992

We were coming back from our bush village Friday when we noticed a crowd gathering in a field outside another village. All of a sudden a man on horseback went into a wild charge toward us. We thought it was a show, like at festivals when the old guys do that, get on their steeds and go into a blazing dusty gallop towards the crowd, raring up and coming to a scary, bouncing stop at the last minute. (Usually, that is: we have also seen the stop part fail.) The man galloped right on by us, though, only eventually coming to a rickety stop, struggling as if to control a spooked horse. Then several men started running towards us, shouting. I heard only two words, doctor and stabbed. They were all kind of crazy and confused, and we had to sort out whether in fact there was a living victim and they wanted me to come. There was, and they did. We urged the Land Rover over the parched corrugated field and came to where the crowd was gathered around a young man lying curled on the ground, blood drizzling from his mouth and nose, his pants soaked scarlet, a neat 5 cm stab wound through his back on the left side. Someone had taken his shirt and cinched it around the thorax in an effort to stanch the flow of blood. Women wailing, men shuffling about in confusion. The young man could talk, but he was breathless and coughing out sticky blood; his blood pressure was scraping bottom and his chest on the left side crackled under my stethoscope. His lung had been pierced, but I couldn't tell whether the heart or the tissues around it had been nicked. We lifted him into the Land Rover and Bello took off like a jet pilot over our treacherous road—I was fearing at this point as much for the vehicle as for the victim. Upon arrival in Kolofata we spent a couple of hours scrubbing and patching him up and propping up his blood pressure, and mostly hoping for the best since we had little at our disposal with which to do much more. He had a rocky go of it all Friday afternoon, but by night he started to settle down and Saturday nothing bad happened. Today he's up a little, and things are looking hopeful.

Oh yes, his crime? He, a Mandara, and his sheep walked across that empty field which belonged to a fellow villager who happened to be a Shuwa.

The God in Kolofata

Sunday, 22 March 1992

A baby—a year old I guess—from Kolofata got measles last week. His parents didn't bring him and didn't bring him and didn't bring him until he could hardly breathe anymore. Then the mother gathered him in her arms and carried him up the hill and sat down in my office and I watched him die. And I was thinking here I am a doctor watching a child from my own town die of what would have been curable complications of an entirely preventable disease. A whole life, body and soul, gone, poof. The mother pressed her hands over the child's eyes, stood up and walked away.

We have vaccinated against measles every blessed day in Kolofata for the past 365 days, and people have known it and dozens if not hundreds have been too lazy—it doesn't cost a cent—to bother bringing their kids. And now they are sick—anyway, it is the will of God—and the tears are flowing and there is no consolation. And seeing the senseless waste of life tires me even more than the hours of hard work.

We are not eating much or sleeping much—the time just isn't there—which does not give much of a boost to my pleasant bedside manner. Anxiety plagues me every time I dare to sit or—God forbid—lie down, for the moment I do, I am under the impression that neon lights go on all over town saying, "She's free— quick! Go knock at her door!" And so they do.

Saturday, 4 April 1992

It is Ramadan. AA is here and in high spirits. We've had some good time to chat with him and he as usual has demonstrated much personal concern for our welfare. He sent over beautiful cloth for us both—it is tradition to give family members cloth for Ramadan—and "dug up" a video player and TV for us to use (the ambassador previously had sent up some cassettes) and mentioned the other day that he intended to do everything he can do to get us to stay. We did not say so at the time, but staying is not the problem as much as staying sane—and that seems to be getting increasingly difficult.

Remember in Naka the woman who had her nose bitten off by an irate husband? Yesterday we had a woman who'd had her ear bitten off in the morning. Chomp. She'll not have to worry about losing the odd earring down the drain any more. The chief of police was investigating the crime and was hopelessly hung up on the fact that the bitten off piece—the whole outside third of the auricle, lobe included—was nowhere to be found. The big question was whether the offender had swallowed it—the woman said yes—or if not where exactly it had gone, for an ear does not just disappear like that. He is waiting for my report.

2 June 1992

Hi. Quick, very quick, note, which will be, I think, the last you will receive before we see each other again.

Pulled away from my cup of coffee this morning by the nurse on duty reporting the arrival of a woman—she turned out to be no more than a girl, 14 years old if even that—who had been slashed in the head last night by her co-wife. Went up to the hospital and found this girl there, lying on the table, her head chopped open, bone fragments and little white blobs of brain tissue hanging out of the wound. The left side, temporo/parietal. She was conscious, though sleepy. Understood clearly but was unable to speak, only sounds coming out like someone who had had a stroke. (For her, a stroke would have been a picnic.) I checked her out, was sure she was stable, the bleeding controlled, and told the family that really this was something that should be handled by the provincial hospital in Maroua, not us, if they could possibly afford to take her there. Family conference followed, men mumbling softly to one another. It is rare that patients are willing to go anywhere else once they have come this far, and so it was in this case. The conference did not last long. The older man came over to speak. An uncle or something. (Neither father nor husband anywhere to be found.) "The God in Maroua is no different from the God in Kolofata," he said. "Will you do what you can do?" So we did what we could, and now she is in the hands of the God of Kolofata, and we will see what he/she/it has planned for this girl. To survive will require a small miracle.

Happy Father's Day, Dad. I saw a picture in a magazine today of an old Underwood typewriter, and I smiled. I love you and thank you.

Soon, then.

Part II

*What do we live for, if it is not to make
life less difficult for each other?*

George Eliot

MYRA AND I took our first home leave during the summer of 1992. We spent much of that leave, as we would spend all our leaves, raising awareness and trying to generate financial support for our work. As soon as we returned to Kolofata we set about expanding the old building on the hill and constructing a new pavilion beside it. The expanded building would be for deliveries and inpatients, who for now were still being housed in the old hospital at the other end of town. The new pavilion would be for consultations, laboratory, and pharmacy.

Inauguration of the two new buildings was being planned for June 1993. There would be a grand ceremony officiated by the minister of health and attended by the US ambassador to Cameroon. We were impatient for this to happen, and mostly we were impatient for outpatient care and inpatient care to be brought together in one place on the hill. We wanted to stop talking about "the hospital" down below and "the clinic" up above. Only after that happened could the Kolofata Hospital begin to flourish and achieve what we believed to be its destiny.

She Made It Clear That She Had Reached Her Final Destination

Friday, 5 March 1993

Our biggest headache has been trying to control our gov't nursing staff, several of whom have reverted to the old practice of trying to extract substantial sums of money from ignorant patients, clandestinely and under threat. You cannot appeal to their sense of professional pride or integrity, because they have none. You cannot appeal to higher authorities, either administrative or professional, because they all, in some way or other, do the same thing. In fact some of them profit directly from the nurses' blackmail and fraud. So we do all we can to make sure the message infiltrates into the population and hope that the people themselves will eventually put a stop to it. Nothing in development work is as discouraging or depressing as watching the haves continually suck the juice from the have-nots and then get together and cluck and laugh at how shriveled they are.

Shortly before twelve o'clock on a hot night at the end of March, Myra and I were awakened by vigorous knocks at our door. I threw on a dress and opened the door to find a young woman lying in the sand, two others standing beside her.

"She is having abdominal pain," one said. "The water is coming out."

"Wonderful," I muttered under my breath and, knowing too well the answer, asked out loud, "what water?"

"The baby's water."

"Labor?" I asked, hoping stupidly that it was not.

"Maybe," the woman in the red replied. "First baby."

"The delivery room is up there," I said, pointing to the hospital.

They did not budge. The woman on the ground grimaced and groaned softly.

I told them they would have to go to the hospital, but I would just take a look to be sure they had time to get there.

I fetched a glove and knelt to examine the young mother-to-be. As I did, she bore down with a mighty force clearly intended to make it known that regarding this pregnancy she had reached her final destination. The cervix was fully dilated in any case, the baby's head was well down, and before long wet tufts of black hair started to appear.

Myra rustled up a woven mat and a couple of clean-enough cloths, and we readied the emergency delivery kit we kept on hand. We had used it many times, but never in our own backyard. Everything then seemed to happen in slow motion, and I felt as if I were watching from above: the black night, the bare bulb above our back door, musicians drumming and piping outside the compound walls, my knees sunk in the sharp sand, the two women hovering and watching and quietly coaching, the mother straining against gritted teeth, the molded head easing ever so slowly into my palms. It was a beautiful, peaceful birth, and when it was over and the baby swaddled and the mat cleaned up, we watched the threesome amble off into the darkness from which they had come, one of them carrying the newborn girl, a whole other life just begun.

A few days later I had to go up to the hospital after dark to retrieve a paper I had forgotten to bring home. When I arrived, I noticed a clump of people sitting on a bench under a tree, others standing around them. The nurse on duty was nowhere to be found, but I presumed he had gone home for dinner and would be back shortly. Annoyed that the sick person in this little group had come to the hospital at night instead of during consulting hours, I made no effort to find out what their problem might be. No one among them attempted to appeal or signal to me either, so I walked past them, retrieved the paper I needed, returned to the Land Rover, and got in. Just as I started the engine, a woman came running over.

"The child," she said, "please."

"Bring him first thing tomorrow morning," I said. "I will see him then."

"No," she said, "please. He is not talking."

The crowd was getting agitated now, and I was feeling less than content for many reasons. I got out of the car and walked over to the bench, running through my mind the differential diagnosis of a child not talking: cerebral malaria, meningitis, sepsis . . .

"When did it start?" I asked as I approached the old father, or maybe grandfather, who sat crying with a boy in his arms. The child looked to be two and a half or three years old.

"Just now," they all said.

It was impossible to know when to believe this very typical response. Probably there were times when it was true. More often it was the standard response given when people did not want to be chided for having waited so long before seeking medical help.

A glimpse at the limp body was enough to tell me we were in trouble. I rushed the father into my office and under the light saw that the boy was not breathing. The father by now was sobbing. The crowd had crushed into the office after us, and people were getting more and more upset. I was fairly convinced the child was already dead, but when I put my stethoscope to his heart, I was stunned and thrilled to hear a beat.

"What happened?" I demanded, desperate for information that might help me decide what to do next. "Has he been sick? Feverish? Did he fall? Did he take something?"

No one admitted a thing. He had been fine, perfectly fine, and then suddenly he wasn't, and that was as much as anyone would say.

Grabbing the boy from his father's arms, I gave his chest a gentle shake. Again stunned and thrilled, I saw him take a breath. Another gentle shake yielded a whimper. A third and he took it upon himself to cry.

Incredulous stares accompanied this progression, and my own was among them. What was magic if not this?

In short order the story came pouring out from all sides: the boy had been playing, and the son of that man over there had knocked him down, and he had lost consciousness, and then when they got here, he had just stopped breathing. I figured that must have been only seconds before I saw him, for his recovery was quick.

The women regained their composure, the father dried his tears. I instructed someone to sit at his bedside all night and nudge him awake every half hour or so, just to be sure, and with words of gratitude and glee they trudged off, the whole clump of them, and I went home, feeling good.

As our work progressed, it gathered more and more attention from people from farther and farther afield. Not all of the attention was favorable. The medical establishment felt threatened by a model of health care that gave prime of place to patients, not doctors, and to care based in communities, not hospitals. Bizarre rumors started to circulate: that we were challenging the Ministry of Health, refusing to collaborate with authorities, treating people for free in order to win naive hearts and minds for some unstated nefarious purpose, murdering patients.

We understood, sadly, that it was not in the interest of the political opposition to see anything associated with anyone in government succeed. As was the case in many of the nascent democracies of Africa, the notion of a loyal opposition was undeveloped in Cameroon. The political opposition saw its role as that of destroyer whose duty was to discredit and undermine existing structures before pouncing and plundering when the walls came tumbling down. "You see," Amadou Ali would ask, "where your 'democracy' has gotten us?"

Myra and I were of no importance, but our area was a politically pivotal one, and we and our work were strongly associated with Ali, a key member of the national administration in a country where political fights had no room in the ring for the good of the people.

In development work, if it is succeeding, there will always be those who wish to sabotage efforts for personal or political gain. Improvement means change, and change is not change if it does not get people upset. Faced with resistance, we resolved to just keep moving ahead, see how far we could get, while being ready at all times to pull up stakes and leave if circumstances forced us to go.

For this reason, we were anxious to get the building finished and functioning without further delay. If the forces stacked against us succeeded in tugging the rug out from under us, we could at least go knowing that we left behind the basic tools needed for the service to survive.

Wednesday, 5 May 1993

The wind blows like a heat blast from a furnace, whipping dry dust everywhere. You come in from a morning in bush and feel like you've been sandblasted. Yesterday we got caught in a dust storm. Visibility was about ten feet, and the "road" became impossible to follow. The Land Rover was full of people and we had to roll up the windows and close the vents. The sweat flowed in rivulets from everyone.

Then at about 7:30 we had just settled down with our mango—dinner these days, as it is too hot to want anything else—when there came a knock at the door. The husband of a woman in labor. We had left her and the nurse on duty at the hospital about half an hour before. The woman had just delivered, it seemed. By herself. The nurse had gone away just after I'd left him, though he was the only one on duty and knew the woman was about to deliver. Something about he was hungry. I grabbed my bag and Myra grabbed the delivery kit and off we went. Imagine my astonishment when I walked into the delivery room (closet, cubbyhole, call it what you will) and found the woman sitting on the floor in a pile of sand, her body from the waist down covered with sand, the new baby lying between her legs [and] covered head-face-belly-cord-to-toe with sand. There was thick dirt everywhere. Myra and I stopped in our tracks. The mother-in-law was crouched on the floor by the mother. Finally I [brought] myself to ask why exactly—my voice as gentle as I could get it to be—they had shoveled dirt on the baby. And the mother. And all over the room. Well, it was just custom, the mother-in-law answered, to clean things up that way. That was as much understanding as I gained. I asked her if she would mind if we washed it all off now, and no, no, she wouldn't mind at all. So we cleaned the cord and clamped it and cut it and took the baby out for his first bath. It was not easy to get the caked dirt off his eyes and lips. Sometime during all this the useless nurse came back ("Geez, I didn't even get to eat.") and immediately launched a wordy tirade about the stupidity of these people who know nothing and do dumb things such as he has never seen before on the face of this earth and why don't they start sending their children to school. Useless to point out to him that if they started sending their children to school—and maybe, just maybe, they know this—they, the children, would risk turning out like him, and God help the country then.

Came back [home] to find a woman of about 50 bleeding on our doorstep, a 9 cm ragged gash [cutting] through her forehead to her skull. The skull intact. Some boy had attacked her because her goat had been drinking water from his pot. I fixed her up.

The final stages of the building were more exasperating and time-consuming than bigger, earlier stages had been. One night at nine the painters called to inform me that they were out of paint, something that could be bought only in Maroua, one hundred rugged kilometers away. As usual, and regardless of how hoarse I got trying to teach workers to order things *before* they were finished, no one from the highest up to the lowest down uttered a peep until the last molecule of a consumable had been consumed. This was as true of paint, lumber, iron rebar, and electrical wire on construction sites as it was of needles, gauze, paper, and water at the hospital. We could keep a secret reserve of medical supplies hidden out of sight in a hospital cupboard, but the cost of building materials was too high to allow us to hoard what in the end might never be needed. So time and again we ran out of things and had to make an emergency run into Maroua, and each time I ranted.

I have no doubt that I in turn proved exasperating to our construction workers. They thought me unreasonably critical of right angles that measured closer to eighty or one hundred degrees than ninety. They wondered why I lashed out if a blue wall drifted into green because that was the color of Pantex they had left. Every time the painters saw me coming they narrowed their eyes and held their brushes suspended in midair.

When I pointed out a "straight" line that dipped, they explained, "Well, the floor isn't flat there."

When I pointed out paint already falling in great chunks from the ceiling, they explained, "Well, the paint"—paint that they had selected—"you bought was of poor quality."

When I pointed at the dark gray from the window frames dripping and smearing the light gray walls, they moaned, "We'll fix it, we'll fix it."

The plumber put many of his pipes in backward and had to dig them up—along with the painted wall and tiled floor that covered them.

The electrician's cable "didn't quite reach," and his materials cost three times his original estimate.

The standard reply to demands to find a better way of doing something done wrong was a shrug of the shoulders and bluff reassurance, "*Il n'y a pas de problème.*"

At least a painter, plumber, or mason who did a bad job could be replaced. The same was not true of our nurses. Posted by Yaoundé, paid by Yaoundé, ruled by Yaoundé, they were out of our control. They were paid at the end of each month regardless of whether or not they came to the hospital or worked when they were there. All were from elsewhere in the country and of ethnic backgrounds and cultures that had little in common with those of Kolofata. They felt contempt for the local population and did not hesitate to rail about how dirty and stupid the people were.

One morning I asked the nurse who had been on duty the night before why he had not given the inpatients their injections during the night. He looked at me in disgust. "Let them inject themselves," he replied.

Another nurse showed up drunk one afternoon. Pretending he had a machine gun, he paced up and down the veranda shooting everyone he passed.

But miracles happen, and in late June the Ministry of Health announced that it was removing three of our most egregious nurses and sending us six new ones. I rejoiced, though with some reservation: if the six new ones ended up being equally bad, we would only be doubling our trouble.

Sunday, 20 June 1993

[A] boy of about 14 [was] stabbed during the night by another boy of the same age in one of our farthest villages. Right chest, fortunately, but the knife sank clear through a rib and into the lung. When he breathed, a wheezing sound

issued through the wound, and when I swabbed it with antiseptic the liquid bubbled right back at me. The right shoulder was also cut up. I was working on him when a neighbor woman and her entourage rushed in panic-stricken, carrying a convulsing 3 year old. Myra was dispatched to get him under control, and then not long after, the other boy of the knife fight pair was brought in, he also with a chest wound, though a milder one. All this [was happening] with our regular outpatients piling up, the masons and the electrician wandering in and out, a Boy Scout out digging holes for our saplings, a nurse from one of our health centers coming to get some papers regularized, a TB patient—a driver—who had come for a blood test complaining that his boss would be raging that he was gone so long, a couple of kwashiorkors crying implacably in the waiting room, a Peace Corps representative whom we met with yesterday coming to leave his last messages and take ours away, a woman needing her infected hand drained of pus, a crazy guy (four times my size, with one eye and a big stick) demanding I look at his hurting leg, Myra coming in every once in a while to ask how I'm doing and cheer me on. In short, a typical morning.

As inauguration day approached, we began to receive a flowing stream of sub-dignitaries coming to reassure themselves that everything would be ready in time to receive their bosses. These would include the minister of health, the American ambassador, the governor of the Far North, television cameras, and a bevy of reporters, administrators, and politicians. Some of our preinauguration visitors came already planning to praise, others to criticize. There was a note of panic in the voices of some of these visitors. I countered them all with "Don't worry about a thing, it will be ready," and then I suggested that if they did not leave us alone to get on with the work, I would be pushing a broom or a paintbrush into their hands. Amadou Ali came two days before the event and was one of the few not to express doubt that we would pull it together in time.

All who had been invited to come came, and many uninvited curiosity seekers tagged along. One woman from the US Embassy said to me, "I've heard so much about Kolofata, I had to see for myself."

Thousands of people from Kolofata and surrounding villages were gathered around the new buildings. Banners flew, musicians drummed and piped, smartly dressed military men and women stood at attention. After the mayor's welcoming speech, a representative of Kolofata's elite took the microphone.

Thursday, 1 July 1993

He spoke eloquently, and there was a paragraph for us, as he cited some of the struggling we have been through. And he added, "For all of this we can offer only one word: Continuez"—which brought a warm cheer from the crowd. I spoke next. I ended in Kanuri, handing the building over to the people and asking them to keep it well. They whooped and clapped and were thrilled. Those few seconds of the ceremony would be talked about for days. I think hearing their own language spoken by a foreigner over an amplifier to an audience of foreign (for anything which is not Kolofatan is foreign) dignitaries and national TV—I think that little thing made them prouder than the gorgeous building, the visiting VIPs and even the special polish that had been put on their town in the preceding days. The American Ambassador followed with her speech, and the Minister closed dryly. We had the ribbon cutting ceremony. Then I led the entourage on the grand tour. A distillation of comments: It's so animated . . . The people must feel at home here . . . I never thought it would be ready . . . It's amazing what you have been able to do with so little . . . And the Minister, hearing that the new building cost 7½ million francs shook his head and said, If I gave 80 million francs to get a building like this put up, we would never see anything. And the other fairly common comment from some of the more establishment city types: It's really very—different. Oh yes, I always agreed heartily, this is not a typical hospital.

Once the brouhaha of the inauguration ceremony and feasting died down, it was back to work as usual, and work as usual was endless. Nothing seemed as fleeting as a peaceful Sunday morning; it was my favorite time of the week. When the weather was fine, I would sit outside at a table under the trees, writing or reading, enjoying the shade, the breeze, the birds, and the squeals of children playing in the street just over our wall. On such mornings a motorcycle carrying a sick child or an injured farmer or a pregnant woman rumbling up to our gate would cause my heart to sink. Rare were the mornings when no motorcycle came, and those were heavenly.

Malaria got worse as the rainy season neared its end. More children presented, and the sick were sicker. Over a forty-hour period at the end of August we received four children under five in coma with cerebral malaria. One had been convulsing nonstop for several hours, another for two days. Three of the four were also seriously anemic.

The coma of cerebral malaria is not a quiet, still one. Fever rages on and off. The body is drenched in sweat and then dries and becomes parched and scorching hot as the temperature rises again. If the child is stimulated, even lightly touched, his mouth clamps shut, his teeth sometimes catching his tongue in their vise. Saliva gurgles in the throat. For days, his brain drags his restless, thrashing body through that dark tunnel where the air is stifling and no light shines. And then . . . And then, if things are going well, after a day or two or maybe three, a relative calm comes at last. The twitchings diminish, the fever spikes fail to climb so far so fast, the tense muscles relax. One day a nurse notices that an injection causes the leg to withdraw gently. It is an almost imperceptible movement, but it is real. This minimal reaction goes on for hours, maybe days, and then at some magical moment a pinch of the skin on the thigh results in the child pulling the whole leg away. A pinch of the skin on the other thigh results in him pulling the other leg away. A pinch of the skin on his arm and then his other arm results in him pulling and pulling, and finally, at last, he opens his eyes and looks at something. He doesn't just stare blindly, he *looks* at something, calmly, patiently, as if waiting for his eyes to bring the target of his regard into focus. And then after a while those eyes slide around and look at someone else's eyes—a mother's, a health worker's— and they hold their gaze for a few seconds before the lids close over them again, and the child falls back to sleep. Anyone witnessing this feels the presence of angels and knows that the wretched battle is won. The room reverberates with sighs of awe and praise for Allah, and one senses hope filling the hearts of other mothers whose unconscious children still lie in their fiery limbo beside them.

I had feared that three of the four would die and had not dared imagine that all would live, but they did.

Saturday, 25 September 1993

We have been into one of those horrendous periods. Myra says, when have we ever not been in one of those horrendous periods, but she is just too tired to remember. I venture reluctantly out of bed every morning knowing it is to face another 24 hours' struggle to keep up with our ever increasing patients, the hundreds of peripheral demands that bombard us every day (car problems, building problems, meetings, staff problems, political shenanigans . . .) and last but not least our own needs of food, water and rest. It is a battle we never come close to winning, but surviving intact to face another day of more of the same is considered a victory of sorts.

The government has posted a young Camerounian doctor to Kolofata to work under me. It would be nice to believe that this was a gesture of goodwill and good faith, and heaven knows we need the help, but the general belief is that it was yet another political move intended to seed trouble. He has supposedly been here for 3 months now, but in that time has put in a total of 11 days—half days, mostly—[of] work, and has caused more than his share of problems already. So we are weary with having to deal with that kind of nonsense on top of everything else. And we also assume that that was the intention of whoever was responsible for shipping him off to us. All we need here—and it doesn't seem to me to be a very lofty or complicated need—is someone who cares about the people. "Teach him," the Minister [of Health] said, "how to behave." As if he knew perfectly well what kind of gem he was sending us. Sure, I said.

The paper I worked on last summer was published by the Transactions of the Royal Society of Tropical Medicine and Hygiene. We have since submitted a sequel which they will also publish if we agree to change some wording regarding Muslims and non-Muslims. Seems suddenly our topic is quite à la mode, what with the Muslim/non-Muslim conflicts flourishing around the world. Our underlying purpose is to point out the powerful effect of culture on health and disease—and thus the necessity of taking cultural differences into account when planning health care or disease control programs. Not a very earthshaking concept in principle, but important in practice. People perceive and think and behave in radically different ways in groups, and these differences have tangible consequences, in our case concerning health. The fact that our two groups happened to be Muslim and non-Muslim was accidental, and given the current world situation, somewhere between the acceptance of the first paper and the second the editors seem to have been piqued by a pang of anxiety. The follow-up paper has to do with differences in infant feeding practices between Muslims and non-Muslims—the former unlike the latter having a tendency to withhold breast[milk] for the first three days, among other differences. One of the reviewers was a well-known tropical paediatrician—he must be a thousand years old by now, for I was reading his books which were already classics when I started medical school—and said, "Excellent paper, and had the results gone the other way I would have no qualms, but given the current political climate could you not find some other way of labeling the two groups?" Has Muslim become a dirty word out there??

As 1993 came to an end, the government took away two more of our worst nurses and sent us three new ones. Two of them looked to be good; the third lived in a state of near-perpetual drunkenness. But for Kolofata, two out of three was excellent, and we cheerfully counted our blessings.

Sunday, 9 January 1994

Our esteemed mayor—previously described to you as a buffoon, I believe, a description I stand by—has been relieved of his responsibilities following an investigation into allegations that he had stolen millions of francs from the community coffers. I was called to appear before the comptrollers, three burly men seated at a long table laden with bulging files. The enquiry was straightforward. One man would open a file and take out a document and ask, "Did the mayor, in the name of the community, give to the hospital in July 1991 the following items: 10 sacks of cement, 100 kg of millet, 20 mats, 5 reams of paper . . ." I would answer no. Another man then would open a file and take out a document and ask, "Did the mayor, in the name of the community, give to the hospital in September 1991 the following items: 4 cartons of soap, a drum of diesel, 120 cartons of cooking oil . . ." And I would answer no. And on and on it went. People like that in places like this never disappear, and he will continue to be an influential force to reckon with (he is the one who has always been against us because we cut into his shady drug business) but at least he slides a notch out of reach.

Wednesday, 19 January 1994

Just after 9 PM and we are beginning what could turn into a nightlong vigil with a noisy lady in labor. [I had] had little sleep last night before being called for another delivery at 5 this morning, [so] this was not in the program for tonight. I came up innocently an hour or so ago to check a child I was worried about—fell out of a tree and banged up his liver—and found the nurse on duty very drunk. He had this woman on the delivery table and was alternately playing with the string around her neck and pinching her lips closed, his fist in her vagina pushing every time she screamed a little louder. I had to pry him off her/ out of her, which was nerve-racking as he is twice my weight and a combative drunk and was not particularly interested in stopping what he was doing. I told the woman to get off the table and start walking, and while the nurse was still trying to get his bearings we marched her over into the other building and locked the doors behind us. So here we are. The nurse wandered over after a while and asked through the window if he could go home and I said that sounded like a good idea.

AA popped in last night—which was why it became a late one for us—and we had an engrossing evening of talk made suddenly and tragically dramatic when a telegram came informing him that 5 of his men had just been killed in an ambush. The men had been part of an operation designed to capture bands of armed robbers that are becoming more and more active, bold and successful in the Extreme-North. The telegram came and AA read it and gave a short stifled agonizing shriek and then he handed it to me and I read first the stark white sheet that said on top Gendarmes Killed and then listed them by rank, 1, 2, 3, 4, 5. Then on the bottom half of the sheet Soldiers Killed, Rank Unknown, 1, 2, 3. The telegram itself explained briefly what had happened. The room was full of family and a couple of gendarmes, and the talk went on for hours.

Sunday, 6 February 1994

Sunday afternoon, and we are trying to squeeze our weekend into a couple of hours. "Hurry up and relax" is our motto these days. You get to the point where the tiniest thing can set you off and even as you overreact you know you are overreacting—or else you under-react and you know you are under-reacting—but you just can't get it right. At times things seem held together with the unstickiest of unsticky glues. And all the pieces lean in their precarious way on you, and although you know you are made of rock you can't figure out how the wind still manages to blow you about as it does.

Friday, 10 June 1994

I once again find myself spending a Friday night at the hospital, this time waiting to see if an aborting woman would kindly stop haemorrhaging. She is being stubborn about it and is sure she is going to die—a heck of an attitude to have in our hospital. I don't think she will. But I wish she'd stop bleeding.

So it is you and I, the hot still night, my fluorescent bulb cutting the darkness, the whirr of the ceiling fan blurring the cries of children over in the children's ward.

You and I and our 6 foot 8 inch cobra. A bunch of boys—8, 10 years old—brought it to the house last night. They had found it in a hole somewhere behind the hospital and they had got out their slingshots and bombarded it to death—they thought, let me add here—and brought it to me because they know we have this neat display at the hospital. Black black, 3–4 inch diameter. Six feet 8 inches long. We measured it. Checked up close the distinguishing features to be sure it was a cobra. Took a few pictures. Myra lay down next to it to demonstrate its length. Don't, she said, take my feet, but I think I did. I sat on the step with it curling around me. It was a gorgeous specimen. Marvelously intact. And then, *well, didn't it start to move. Just the tail at first, and I said to Myra, No no, it must just be a nervous twitch—See where the spine must be broken? And then, well, didn't he (oops—did my it suddenly become a he?) start to wiggle his back. And on up. The neck, the head. The boys (long gone, their slingshots gone with them) had said he'd been eating some animal when they'd "killed" him and they'd wrestled the animal free afterwards, and I wondered now how hungry he must be.*

Went in to get a broom and I banged him over the head—gently, because I didn't want to wreck it—enough to stun him so we could get him into a box (big box) and pack him into the Land Rover, and [I] drove—rather quickly—up to the hospital. He was still inert so I started injecting him with 95% ethanol. Ho ho ho. Snakes love 95% ethanol. He once again regained consciousness, and his body's sinuous curves went back into motion. Our night guard [Ali], himself some-thing of a lusty drinker, thought this was a delightful thing to behold. "L'alcool, l'alcool," he extolled. Nevertheless he managed to maintain control of his senses and went to find a big stick with which he held the cobra's head down while I finished injecting. Before I got to the neck [Ali] obligingly gave a few good taps to be sure there would be no more movement. And so the deed was eventually completed. The beautiful thing now lies curled half a dozen times in a covered bucket of alcohol here in my room. We are waiting to locate a jar big enough (we know where one is, but we have to get to Maroua) for him so he can take his place among our growing menagerie.

We took our second leave during the summer of 1994 and returned to Kolofata in early October. I had loved being in America—seeing family and friends, rev-eling in the luxuries of running water, ice cream, clean buildings—but being in Kolofata was another kind of contentment that convinced me I was exactly where I was supposed to be. The rains had been good, and the millet was reaching for the sky. It was nighttime when the Land Rover rolled into town, but a group of teenage boys congregated on the side of the road recognized it as it approached and in unison rose and started clapping. We were welcomed warmly by young and old, none of whom minced words letting us know how terrible it was that we had left them and how pleased they were that we were back.

Having spent the summer with humongous Americans of all ages, I was struck anew by how small and skinny and full of knees and ribs the children in Kolofata were. The sick ones, the ones too weak even to cry, captivated my soul. I held their tiny wounded-bird bodies in my arms and knew and longed to make them know that if they could just hold on a little longer, they would start to feel better.

Monday, 24 October 1994

Nighttime, but sleep eludes me. I spent half the morning in the delivery room going through the intense and grisly process of trying to get a dead baby out of a young woman who was barely old enough to have been pregnant in the first place. Three day labor. She arrived at the hospital exhausted, no longer contracting, her bladder ballooned with two days' worth of urine she hadn't been able to pass. I was hoping that once we emptied the bladder she'd be able to get the baby out without too much pushing and pulling. But no such luck. It was gruesome. And when the lifeless fetid body finally did come out, the smell seemed to penetrate my every pore and stayed with me all day. Still, being Monday it was busy enough and as I went from patient to patient I thought the delivery was not going to bother me. But at the end of the day one runs out of busyness. And every time I close my eyes I am back in that room, pulling and struggling and smelling the smell. The mother is okay. She hardly cared that the baby was dead. She was glad enough to get it out and to find herself still alive, and although she does not know it, she has probably been spared the lifelong curse of a vesico-vaginal fistula, which surely would have been her lot had she not come when she did.

We prepared a duck for Christmas that year, but the highlight of my day was the arrival of a man in his early sixties who had been hit, reportedly accidentally, over the left ear with a metal bar. The ear had not been severed from his head, but it had been sliced neatly in two and required mending. We chatted as I sutured, and he gave me his life story.

He had been born among the Tuperi in the north, but when he was in his twenties, he joined the army and was sent to Yaoundé, where his job was to participate in raids in the bush to recover rifles and other arms from rebel groups.

"Sounds dangerous," I said.

"Oh yes, I was injured three times and lost many comrades. But I was good at it. They gave me ten medals," he chuckled. "Ten."

He tired of army life and after a decade left—he was vague on whether this was with or without permission—and traveled back up north. One day in 1968 he happened to be on the Nigerian side of a border market when Nigerian armed forces, engaged in a conscription drive targeting all fit men, seized him. The Biafra War was raging, the federal government needed fighters, and the generals did not care if recruits claimed they came from Nigeria, Cameroon, or Mars. He was shipped down south and served in the Nigerian army for six years. The war by then had ended, and he used a month's leave to return to Cameroon. Once there he never looked back.

Thinking of the terrain he had covered and the work he had done, I asked, "So how many languages do you speak?"

He counted on his fingers. "Tuperi, Moundang, Kanuri, Mandara, Hausa, Fulfulde, French, English: eight." He paused, looked at the ceiling. "That's all. Some Arabic, a little Massa."

"Did you ever go to school?"

"Never touched a bench," he replied, referring to the table-benches at which elementary pupils sit.

"So what," I asked, "brought you to Kolofata?"

He smiled and threw out his hands as if to embrace the world. "God," he said. "God just brought me here, and here I am."

"Me too," I said, laughing with him as the last knot was tied and the suture end snipped free.

Sunday, 8th January 1995

It was a week for extractions. I don't know about elsewhere, but in Africa primary care docs are forever extracting things: beads from ears, peanuts from noses, specks from eyes, fly larvae from under the skin, babies from wombs. My harvest this week included a finger bone and a 2-inch long thorn. The first belonged to a lady who had suffered an infection some weeks earlier that had consumed the flesh so that the fingertip had completely disappeared and the finger part of the rest of her finger down to the first joint had shrunken away, leaving the bare bone jutting out. The bone was dead, but it hurt where it was still attached to the stump, and anyway it was, she felt, very inconvenient. I hate amputating, I hate pulling teeth, I'm not even terribly keen about intentionally cutting through anyone's skin (although I am fond of the sewing up part). Up on the table she went, and gritting my teeth I set about dislocating the joint and freeing up the offending bone (stealing repeated glances at her scrunched up eyes, asking now and then if she was feeling dizzy or queasy—and feeling rather dizzy and queasy myself) and then after a gentle tug yielded nothing I braced myself and gave one powerful gentle tug—and out the thing came, snug between the jaws of my forceps. She was delighted.

The thorn was less gruesome but more scary because this poor old guy—well, sixtyish, but that beats the life expectancy here by a generous decade—had managed to stab himself through the palm side of the wrist, embedding this wicked toothpick-size thorn perpendicular to and right on top of his radial artery. The one you aim for when the debts pile up too high or the wife leaves you or the kid declares her independence. For all I knew [the thorn] had ragged edges and no qualms about tearing the artery if I didn't treat it with due respect. The thick end was completely hidden. The pointed end was sticking out a millimeter, through the side of his wrist. "Just pull it!" advised the nurse. "Oh God!" I groaned silently, praising same that He had seen fit not to have that nurse on duty alone when this man came in. After incising the other side of his wrist and digging around, I found the thick end and got it clamped in my forceps. The gentle tug (nothing) followed by the powerful gentle tug yielded our quarry. But with a sickening sensation, and our man covered his face with his other hand and squeezed the knuckles over his eyes. I felt like doing the same, but it hardly seemed proper. I looked at the thorn. It had, in fact, a nice barb along its side, and anyone trying to pull it out from its penetrating end would have sliced the artery. I wrapped the invader in a piece of cotton and gave it to him for a souvenir.

In February we started work on a new building that would include offices, a suite for taking and developing x-rays, and smaller rooms for housing patients who required isolation. Fifty tons of cement were delivered, thousands of concrete blocks were fashioned and set out to harden, iron work on windows and doors began, contracts were drawn up, the outline of the foundation was fenced in, and earnest meetings with various groups were held to keep the community engaged. The bustle of progress was invigorating.

Thursday, 2 March 1995

AA is here to celebrate the end of Ramadan au village. We had a very late dinner last night. As it was his first evening in town he was not yet surrounded by the hundreds of minions (well-wishers, favor-seekers) who between this morning and the moment he leaves will be everywhere constantly. His first night in town is usually just family, and I think it is the time he most enjoys.

It is later now, and as expected the compound has been hopping all day. Cars and trucks going in and out, in and out. I could barely negotiate my way out of the courtyard and into the street to go up to the hospital this evening. And then we got back just as the big chief of a neighboring canton and his entourage were pulling up. The chief was dressed in splendid regalia, his hooded, tassled cloak a shiny silver material, a footman carrying his colorfully sheathed, tassled sword. His—the chief's—head was swathed in numerous twists of white turban, and his eyes were shielded by gold-emblazoned black sunglasses. We stood back against the Land Rover, half in awe, half because it didn't seem politically correct to step anywhere near the path of this shimmering personage. But he spotted us (we, too, tend to stick out in a crowd) and greeted us warmly.

The compound and the town have been alive. In the morning we took a walk around until our hands started to go numb from so much greeting and shaking. Everyone is beautiful today, from the babies to the old great-grandfathers. New cloth, shiny earrings and bracelets, starched bright bonnets on the men, new plastic sandals, all the girls' hair tressed in tight neat braids, many of the kids with dime-store sunglasses and wristwatches. Everybody full of beans.

The spitting, most of it, is over for yet another year.

Three days after the Ramadan holiday a woman of about thirty came to the hospital complaining of abdominal pain.

"Are you pregnant?" I asked.

"Yes," she replied.

"How many months?"

"No, no," she answered. "Eight years."

"Oh," I said. "Well, then, how many months since your last period?"

"Now," she said.

"Did it come last month?" I asked.

"Yes."

"Every month every month?"

"Yes."

I considered it prudent to shift slightly my line of questioning. "Have you had any children?"

"One," she said.

"Alive?"

"Yes."

"How old?"

"Twelve years."

"Did you have any others, others who died?"

"No, just this one inside," she said. "I missed my period for three months—that was eight years ago—and then it came again, but the child didn't come out. Even now," she reminded me, "the blood is coming, and the child is just staying there inside."

I palpated her abdomen.

"Yes, there!" she exclaimed. "That is where he is sitting now. But sometimes he moves to the other side."

This, I thought, was truly wonderful. In most of Africa, infertility, even secondary infertility following the birth of one or two children, is a horrid curse. It is shameful for the woman and intolerable for her husband. This was the perfect solution to a difficult problem. General ignorance was such that most people had no trouble believing a pregnancy could last for many years. Marabouts and traditional healers from time to time made this diagnosis, and it was accepted without dispute. As a result, neither the woman nor her husband had to deal with the stigma of infertility. They were pregnant. Things were just moving along a little more slowly than usual.

Keeping the Front Wheels in Front of the Back

Thursday, 13 July 1995

We got into Maroua last Saturday. Every venture out of Kolofata now becomes an anxious affair, as rain could fall at any time and prevent us from getting back into town. But we had some building things to pick up and had to go. We left early and started ticking off our errands. All was well until we got to the hardware market around ten o'clock. The sky started getting grayish on one horizon and before long blackish, and the horizon kept getting closer and closer.

The hardware market consists of a long alleyway lined on either side by shacks opened wide on the alley side. Like a bunch of mini garages. We have our favorite shops—guys who know us and give us good prices and scramble around to find what we need, often running to a distant neighbor's shop and bringing back some obscure piece they themselves didn't happen to have. (You would love these shops, Mom. They are a mess floor to ceiling and always spilling out the front and the sides, if there happens to be any opening there, and all their odds and ends covered in thick dust and grease, and you just never know what treasure you are going to find tucked away in some hidden far corner. You have to look carefully, patiently, your eyes running slowly and systematically over every nut and bolt, every pulley and spring, every length of chain and plasticized cord, every light, every bucket, every knob and handle, every clamp-like thing, every tin of miracle goops and oils and creams, every metal and plastic bit of tubing, every screw.) We were at one of our favorite shops when the sky opened. Wide. It poured and it poured and it poured. Thunder kabooming, lightning flashing. The shack's roof held, but the alleyway got wetter and wetter and finally turned into a river. The shop we were in might have fit [a midsize car], but you wouldn't have been able to get out of the car once you parked it there. It contained: Myra, me, the owner, his head worker, his gofer and four other young men who were simply passing the time that day. This in addition to floor-to-ceiling shelves laden and bending under the weight, a desk and 2 chairs, and larger equipment—sinks, generators, ladders, roof tar—lining the floor and overflowing voluminously into the alleyway. The owner took charge of us and our order of light fixtures, bulbs, lamps, four big aluminum sinks, pieces of pipe, hinges and a door lock—and all the while as he gathered an item, blew off the dust, tied it up if it needed tying up, and added it to the bill, all the while the rain poured and poured and the river of the alleyway rose. It finally started sneaking into the front of the shop and 2 of the young idlers bravely took up brooms and started swishing it out. Swish swish swish, and it flowed back in. Swish swish swish, and it flowed back in. The owner told us to sit and get our feet up and Myra did but I declined, seeing that sooner or later it would be of no use. The water rose, covering our feet, covering our ankles. The boys with the brooms gave up and dedicated themselves to getting the more perishable goods—generators, cardboard boxes—out of the deeper water. A couple of things we needed the owner did not have, so he rolled his pants up and went out into the river under the downpour and ten minutes later came back with the items, dripping. We waited quietly in the shop, the water rising on our legs, I beginning to shiver, Myra beginning to count our millions. The young men settled down and just watched the rain fall and the owner contentedly tallied up the bill—and it was all very much business as usual, the thunder cracking and the lights blinking spastically and the nails and nozzles disappearing under the rising tide. Eventually all was completed, and the owner and his two helpers and one of the young men hoisted our booty on their shoulders and paraded out towards our Land Rover. Myra and I took a few of the smaller things, hitched our dresses up above our knees and ventured out of the flooded shop into the flooded alleyway and marched on slowly, trying not to splash.

The rain stopped soon after we finished in the hardware market, and no rain fell north of Maroua, so we got back into Kolofata that afternoon with no difficulty whatsoever.

Thursday, 24 August 1995

I am happy tonight to be alive and all in one correctly articulated, unbroken piece. I had a meeting at one of our health centers at 9:30. The rain [from the night] stopped and I thought that by the time I had to leave at 9:00 the road would be dry enough to be negotiable. Most of it was. But there is a stretch of almost a kilometer which is pure black mud. Not the kind you get stuck in but the kind that slips like crazy. Not only that, but this particular stretch has 3 culverts over which the road is built up, so there is a ten or fifteen foot drop off either side into a swamp studded with boulders. These challenging obstacles look like mudslides, black and glistening, and they are just wide enough to allow a single vehicle to get over—provided the vehicle is going straight: that is, front wheels in front of back wheels.

Which is the problem, because when you are sliding through muck there is no way anyone can keep his front wheels in front of his back wheels. All the laws of physics are against it. The differential lock is great for getting through thick mud, but greasy slick mud is something else, and I don't find much difference riding with four wheels or two.

I got to the meeting. It was like prancing sideways on a circus horse part of the way, and I was shaking like a leaf when I finally hit semisolid ground again, but I got there. I figured, logically I thought, that [with] a couple of hours of sunshine the road would dry up and I would make it back. The meeting went well. Two hours later I got into the Land Rover, started back and ran right into rain. Heavy rain this time. But short, and it was down to a drizzle when I got to the bad spot. A tanker was parked there, and two cars, [the drivers] knowing they could not make it [across]. I stopped to see what they thought, and they thought I ought to be able to get through.

So I inched forward. Sort of forward. A bit forward, a bit angled, a bit sideways. The urge to brake becomes irresistible, yet that is the last thing you want to do. I inched along, inched along, slip slip slide slide, and got to the run-up of the highest culvert, did a 45° spin and decided that was all I wanted to do. Another 45° would get me over the side, and I got to thinking that I've not enough fat on me to protect many of my bones, and besides, I love that Land Rover. So gingerly I backed down and stopped and turned off the engine and just sat. Waiting. Waiting for what, I wasn't sure. The road to dry out? Another vehicle wanting to try and thus forcing me to try, as that would be the only way of getting out of the way? I didn't know. Waiting just seemed to be the thing to do and so I did. After a while a woman walked by, smiled, greeted, went on. Then a man pushing a motorcycle came and asked me if I had a number 10 wrench and I did so I gave it to him and he worked on his bike for a while and finally got it going, and he gave me back the wrench with a smile and straddled his bike and went on, the motor going but his feet staying on the ground to keep balance.

And then finally the driver of the tanker that was parked back there waddled— waddled, because that is the only way you can walk through mud—by and asked if I was going to try again. No, I said, not now. He looked at the road, gauging it; he looked at the Land Rover, gauging it. It's a light vehicle, he said; you should be able to do it. You in 4-wheel drive? Yes, I said. You try it in 1st? he asked. Yes, I said. You try it in 2nd? he asked. No, I said. In 2nd, he said, you shouldn't slide as much.

I have a lot of respect for these tanker drivers. They have years of experience driving rickety mammoth vehicles over treacherous roads under terrible conditions. They also tip over, slide off bridges, burrow into impossibly deep muddy craters, and burn up with great regularity. But this guy inspired confidence (also, he was Camerounian, not Nigerian or Chadian like most of them) so I asked him if he wanted to give it a try. He hesitated. Wry smile. Looked at the road, looked at the Land Rover. Then said okay, he would try. He knocked some of the mud off his feet. I moved over, he got in, I showed him the gears and the pedals. Okay, he said. And ever so slowly slowly slowly we moved forward. Sort of forward. A little sideways, a little forward, a little sideways, a little forward. We climbed the culvert, and at the peak, the fifteen foot drop a few inches away, we skidded. I did find myself saying a little prayer, thanking God for all the good times. We skidded, but then, with the gentlest touch on the wheel he pulled us back around again. The driver I mean. Or God. At that point I was not concerned with petty distinctions. He got us over the culvert and down the other side and then he went ahead and got us to the end of that bad stretch, which I was very happy to let him do. And then he stopped and said, There, I think you'll be fine now. He opened the door and got out, and I thanked him and shook his hand, and he smiled and then bowed and turned to walk back to his truck.

—All of which explains why I am here and able to finish this letter, lucky you.

I am well. Hope you are well. Drive carefully.

I love you.

E

I Am Counting on You, Should God Turn Out to Be Muslim

MAMADOU WAS A marabout, a man in his late twenties, and the first insulin-dependent diabetic I treated in Kolofata. He was calm and soft spoken, short in stature, always pristine in his white cotton *gondora*. At first, the idea that he required a white man's—let alone a white woman's—medicine to stay alive was repugnant to him. It was even more repugnant to the elder marabouts, for whom Mamadou was a prized protégé. We had to wrench him from death's jaws several times before they and he grudgingly accepted his fate.

He took his insulin, kept his appointments faithfully, and remained in good health for a long time. Then one day he came down with dysentery. After trying spiritual and traditional medicine to no avail, he came to the hospital. He was very weak by then, and I recommended admission, but he declined, saying it would not look good to his students. So I gave him medicine for his dysentery and told him to come back in two days if he was not better. Two days came and went, and I was happy not to see him, assuming that meant he was improving.

On a Saturday evening five days later, I left the hospital and was just about to pull the Land Rover into our courtyard when a friend of Mamadou's came running toward us, signaling us to stop. He seemed excited and I was sure he was wanting to tell us that Mamadou was doing well.

This was not the case. "Mamadou is not well at all," he said, supplication in his eyes and agitation in his voice. "Come see."

"What do you mean?" I asked, anger mingling with fear. "I told him to come back to the hospital if he wasn't feeling better, and he didn't come back."

"The old marabouts forbade him to go. They made him stop taking his medicines, even his insulin. They don't understand."

"Well," I said, "Mamadou does. I will not go to his house. But if you take him to the hospital, I will go see him there." I looked past him, stared with despair at the timeless, endless sand.

The friend asked to be forgiven.

"Ask God, not me, for forgiveness." Already I grieved for the gentle soul and wasted life.

Instead of going home, I drove around the block, killed some time, and then turned up Mamadou's street. I drove slowly. All was quiet. Mamadou's compound looked deserted. Only one old woman sat in the courtyard, and she frowned at us somberly, neither beckoning nor otherwise acknowledging our presence. I slowed to a crawl. No one came out; no one signaled, though I knew the people inside could hear the Land Rover's motor. Realizing with miserable regret that they were prepared to sacrifice Mamadou on their altar of pigheadedness, I shifted gears and drove on.

I entered our compound and went into the house, prepared and ate dinner, and all the while awaited a call. An hour passed, another half hour.

At last the friend appeared at the back door. "Mamadou is at the hospital. Will you come?"

"What took you so long?" I asked. I went. Mamadou was in dire distress. His skin was dry as paper. His teeth were like chalk. All his energy was devoted to the task of getting air into and out of his chest. He could talk, but his words were unintelligible. His heart clicked strangely. His belly was sunken, and the skin of it was thick and doughy.

We fretted for forty-eight hours as his body struggled to sort itself out. In the end it did, and within a week he was spending the evenings sitting on the ward veranda surrounded by boys he was teaching to become marabouts, all lounged on pillows and rugs, happily fingering prayer beads. Every time I saw him I felt a gush of relief. On the day of his discharge I wished him health and a long, long life.

"For I am counting on you," I said, "should God turn out to be Muslim."

He nodded, smiled shyly, and left.

Wednesday, 17th January 1996.

We are having unending problems with door handles. In the two big wards we finally took all the inner workings of all the locks out and left the door handles in place only for show. None of the doors now can latch shut—which means that no one can accidentally find himself inside or outside a closed door and experience that terrible panic of not knowing how to open it. There are many other hazards of doors which are not at first obvious to people who are accustomed to dealing with them. Many people who come to our hospital are seeing real doors that open and close for the first time in their lives. And many have this knack of closing the door on their hand when they leave my consulting room. Even of those who have some practical experience with doors, few have ever seen doors on the inside of a building. Hence doorways seem to be easily ignored—or at least, their dimensions seem to be easily miscalculated. I cringe whenever I see a woman with a baby slung on her hip making for my doorway. His head! His head! I am always pleading as I lunge to get a hand on the doorjamb—usually succeeding just milliseconds after the KLUNK *. The new building still has its door handles. Functioning door handles. But they are taking a beating and they will not last. Yesterday evening as I finished my rounds I found one lying forlornly on the verandah—yanked off in someone's fury.*

Sunday, 21st. While we're on the subject of haute technologie, it is worth covering the other problem: of the scale. I have in my consulting room a scale, an ordinary bathroom scale (well, not quite ordinary, as the readings are in your choice of kilograms or stones). Few people have ever seen a scale or have any idea how to get on it and are wary of what it will do (collapse? vibrate? roll away? rise up? tickle their feet?) when they do get on it. An order to "get on the scale" as often as not results in the patient going to sit down on it. No, no, I say, stand on it. This provokes a look first of disbelief then, when the order does not change, of reluctant compliance. The patient grabs on to something—the chair, the window frame, me—and steps cautiously up onto this machine. One foot. Come on, come on, I say. Both feet: here and here. I do my best to show the patient exactly where to put his feet—praying he does not break the window frame as he grapples—and in spite of this, one foot always lands smack on the little plastic window meant to reveal his weight. There follows the difficult task of getting him to shift—I have the impression he feels as though he is standing in a rowboat in choppy seas. All of this takes an enormous amount of time and admirable perseverance on the part of the heroic doctor—who eventually and with a sigh of relief extends a hand to help the poor soul replant his feet on terra firma.

Wednesday, 31 January 1996

The month of Ramadan—those 29 days we all just love—is a week down, three to go. Hack hack hack, spit spit spit. We have decided at last to throw all patience and cultural tolerance to the wind this year and really light into anyone spitting—at least within the confines of our hospital kingdom. Apart from it being simply disgusting, there is too much tuberculosis around these days to turn a blind eye to the habit. We are preaching and chastising with a vengeance, and

I am prepared to go head to head, chapter and verse, with any marabout who tries to tell me the Quran forbids the faithful to swallow their saliva. I have won the nurses over to my side and like many converts they are now fiercer than I in going after anyone who even looks like he is thinking of spitting. They get particularly annoyed at those who carry around little plastic bags or pouches of sand, spit into these all day long and then at the end of the day just drop [them] on the ground in front of the hospital for the groundsman to clean up in the morning. Every morning our grounds are littered with plastic packs of sand and spit.

You will remember my telling you several weeks ago about an anaemic lady brought in one evening and pulled from the brink with the help of a transfusion from her husband. Having none of the usual causes of anemia I suspected a bone marrow problem but hoped it might be temporary—as due, perhaps, to some toxic concoction, medicinal or otherwise, that she had taken at home. With the beginning of Ramadan, the family was anxious to have her back home (the women are required to work hard during Ramadan, all day preparing the feasting that goes on all night) and although I was not keen to discharge her, she was feeling better and assured me she would go home to rest, not work. She was discharged, and a couple of days later she was carried back in much the same state she had been in when we first received her. This time I knew her outlook was grim. She was my age, and she was accompanied by 3 sisters—two younger and one quite a bit older. The youngest had recently miscarried, the middle sister's blood did not match Fatouma's, and so I took a unit from the eldest sister, who gave with abundant joy.

We were not sure Fatouma was going to hang on for us to get the blood drawn and the transfusion going—she was pulling for every breath and suffering terrible chest pains—but she did, and the transfusion slowly settled her down. I knew how temporary would be the relief [but] I could not share my thoughts and expectations with her or the family—because after all there was still, as there always is, that tiny grain of hope, that maybe by some miracle her body would find its way to making its own red cells again—and so the ensuing days were spent trying to concentrate on and soothe the little things that came up. The sore throat. The backache. The insomnia. The crushing chest pains came back. There was no family member left to give blood, and I did not push hard for them to find another donor. We had known Fatouma for years, ever since we helped rescue her skinny crippled tubercular son Souleyman—he is 16 now, tall and fit, a young man already, and he carries a long knife sheathed around his waist and his herder's staff in his hand. She had spent the many weeks of his hospitalization cheerfully caring for him. She had a smile for everyone, and she called me Madame in her high Fulani voice whenever she spoke to me. And during her own illness, right to the end as her oxygen-starved heart screamed within her, she never changed. "Madame, it is here," and she would take my hand and place it against the bony ribs where her pain was most intense.

On the morning of her last day I found her sitting propped up in bed, and she smiled—a flash of hope! Why is there always that bloom before the end? Her remaining strength ebbed quickly over the course of the day, and by afternoon she and her sisters—for the first time, I think—understood that hope was gone.

The husband had gone back to the village two days earlier, so the older sister came as I was finishing my last patients and asked if I would carry them home. They piled their mats and pans [into the Land Rover], and the two younger sisters climbed in the back space and the older sister sat in the back seat with Fatouma lying, her head on her sister's lap, sighing softly with each breath. The village was 20 km away, through several other villages, over rocky roads and foot paths, down a steep bank and across a wide sandy river bed—there were no tracks of any vehicle, even a bicycle, and I imagined the Land Rover getting stuck in the deep sand, and the sun was going down.

Before we reached the village, Fatouma died. The sound of an approaching motor drew everyone from their huts, so that by the time we arrived many people were standing about staring anxiously in silence. Suddenly I heard a woman speak Fatouma's name, and then another woman say something else, and then awareness set in like a fog and the wailing, the wild wailing began. Even before we stopped, the older sister was gesturing sternly to calm people down, but they paid her no heed. We pulled up to Fatouma's hut and the villagers gathered round. One young woman came to my window and shouting madly like all the others struck me repeatedly on the shoulder—not in anger but in helpless grief— saying over and over again, "My sister, my sister, my sister." As the men removed Fatouma from the car I looked out the passenger window and saw Souleyman standing there, mute and still. Our eyes met once, and he looked away. The car unloaded, I left, following my own tracks along the silent paths. She had such grace, right to the end and in spite of all her pain. Her youngest is two, a lively boy named Malloum.

The Father of the Husband Ate Her

THE NEWS THAT greeted us after our 1996 leave was that Amadou Ali had been promoted to general secretary of the presidency, a role roughly equivalent to a US president's chief of staff. He was pleased, so we were pleased and hoped the new job would give him the chance to use his considerable talents and vision to lead the country in a more ubiquitous sense than he had been able to do as minister of defense.

What the new job did not do was shorten his workday. He routinely labored from four in the morning until eleven at night, and his dining table was simply another desk. He seldom enjoyed a meal alone with his family, as there were always others, come to present a problem or seek a favor, around the table. He could not return home at night without finding a crowd from different parts of the country waiting for him. He thrived on that pressure and attention, but there were limits, and we worried that these were being surpassed with increasing frequency.

Yet the country and Africa were in such need of leaders of his caliber, and he knew it, and he refused to let up.

Thursday, 16 January 1997

Tuesday evening we had just finished eating at 7:00 and were about to settle down to some reading and writing when there was a knock at the door. The nurse on duty had sent a note saying that he had just received a woman at term, in labor and unconscious. I grabbed Myra and my bag and up we went. A middle-aged woman [was] lying on the table. Mother of 8, with 2 others who had died. She [had been] well until that afternoon when she started having abdominal pains and breathing strangely, and then she collapsed. On further questioning it turned out that she hadn't eaten much for two days—so she must not have been feeling entirely well for a least two days—and her waters had broken five days earlier. She was conscious when I examined her, but in dire distress. High fever, heart pounding, blood pressure scraping bottom. I am pretty good with lung sounds, but hers were peculiar, and she had wheezing audible through the stethoscope. She was breathing faster than a newborn baby, the chest pumping pumping pumping up and down and up and down and up and down. Every time I listened to her chest she was annoyed almost, saying the pain was not there but in her belly. Her belly contained a dead baby. The cervix was open 7 cm and the head was well down, but there was no fetal heart to be heard. The uterus seemed to be doing its job. There was no sign of internal or external blood loss. But the baby was dead and maybe had been dead for days and [if] the uterus was infected I feared the infection had seeped into her blood. And on top of that some catastrophic event had happened that afternoon or evening. An embolus, maybe, of infected amniotic fluid that lodged in her lungs and triggered the respiratory distress and peculiar lung sounds. We put up a drip and got antibiotics running into her and gave her a bolus of heavy-duty dextrose—her blood sugar was also perilously low—and we got the vacuum ready. I kept monitoring her vital signs, and every increment in the right direction was cause for hope. False hope. How many times during that long night did we feel that mean twinge of false hope.

She calmed down somewhat. Far from entirely, but somewhat. She was able to drink and talk a little. By ten o'clock she was fully dilated and I asked her to push, not thinking that she would have the strength to do so. But she did, and we pulled out the putrid cadaver. That, at least, was over. Twinge of false hope. I pressed on the uterus. Huge gush of blood. Placenta going nowhere. We gave her injections to contract her uterus, and the uterus contracted but the placenta remained stuck. Within minutes it was clear that our worst fear was going to be realized: the blood that had come out was not clotting. Her blood, poisoned by the infection or deranged by an embolus (or both), was not going to clot. She continued to bleed, so I had to go in and manually detach and remove the placenta. This was done and it looked like the bleeding was going to slow down. Twinge of false hope. Her blood pressure [came] up, she relaxed, her fever had come down. I'll be home, I thought, by midnight.

We had taken blood from an 18 year old son and that was running into her, and I was thinking maybe it hadn't even been absolutely necessary to do that.

And then the black curtain dropped. The bleeding picked up. I clamped down on her uterus but every time I let go for a minute and then clamped again it was like wringing a sponge. And then her veins started leaking, as though they were made of mesh. She had IVs running in both her arms, and they kept blowing up. We'd take them out and scout around for another vein and get into it and a few minutes later it, too, would blow up. There was blood everywhere. And the dead baby wrapped in a puce cloth on the side table, and the putrid placenta in a basin on the floor, and the woman, fading now from consciousness, lying on cloths soaked head to toe in her blood. I had drawn another unit of blood—from the husband, who also matched—and it was running into a last precious vein. But all was futile. Her breathing changed from breaths to gasps, her lower jaw thrust forward as it does during that final reaching for air. She died. And the awful wailing began. It continued and rang out in that quiet night in that wilderness on our hill, going on and on like air raid sirens that go on and on even though you know there can be no one left in town who hasn't heard and understood them. We carried her into the back of the Land Rover and laid her dead baby beside her, and I drove her home. It was some time after two.

Everyone has his own way of explaining the tragedy. I do not think this death was avoidable, at least not by the time she got to us and not with the tools we have to work with, and I think it was due to a coagulopathy secondary to a dead infected fetus and probably an embolus. Our people have a different explanation. I asked someone today what the belief was in town concerning this woman's death. I quote: "It was sorcery. The father of the husband ate her." It seems this is the fourth wife this husband has lost, and the conclusion was obvious to all.

Tues, 28 Jan. 1997

A first-time mother was transferred to us from one of our health centers because she was young and small and progressing poorly. The fetus was dead before she reached us, but her pelvis looked big enough to allow her to deliver if she did some serious pushing when the time came. I told the husband that the baby was not alive, and he didn't especially care; all he wanted was for it to be born and for his wife to be okay. I didn't tell her, for fear of discouraging her when she needed all her strength. She would know soon enough. She was chipper for being in so much pain, and when the time came she pushed with determination. Every once in a while she would lie back exhausted and gasp that she was too tired, she couldn't do any more. And I would laugh and say, Okay, then, I'll go and come back when you're ready, and she would immediately take a deep breath and push. I suppose she was fifteen years old. A very little fifteen. She was feeling pressure on her rectum as the head came down and she reached out and drew me to her—there was a male nurse in the room with me—and whispered helpfully and with insistence, "It's coming out my bottom!" No, no, I said, that's just the pain; the baby's right where he's supposed to be. "But look again," she whispered, more emphatically still, "it's coming out my bottom!" Fortunately the head was crowning and I directed her hand to touch the bulging mat of curly hair and she was reassured and so delighted she gave one last heroic push and out he came. She raised a clenched fist and thanked me over and over again, and when she was settled back down I had to tell her that the baby was dead. She looked over and it registered and she started to cry softly, and the nurse quickly cut her off with a scold, "Ha! None of that. You will have more." And she looked at him, reflected for a second, and dried her tears.

In early June parliamentary election results were announced, and a romp by the party in power was confirmed. Party leaders maintained that the overwhelming victory was a clear sign that the people were satisfied. Opposition leaders maintained that their defeat was a clear sign that fraud in favor of the victors was rampant.

Chatting with me at the hospital, a visitor from Mora said that in the *pays des blancs* nothing like this would happen. "The party in power does not hold on to power even after an election."

I informed him that Canada had recently held an election and that the ruling party had in fact retained its majority.

He sat back sharply, slapped his thighs, and exclaimed, "Ha! So even in the *pays des blancs* elections are marred by fraud!"

Wondering what I had said that he misunderstood, I looked at him curiously and asked him why he said that.

"Well, I thought you said that in Canada the party in power won the election."

"Yes."

"Then"—and now it was his turn to look curiously at me, wondering, perhaps, if I really did not see the obvious or if I was pulling his leg—"there must have been fraud."

"But what if a population is generally pleased with its elected government?" I proposed. "Can it not honestly reelect those representatives?"

He shook his head. "People always want change. Let me give you an example. Let's say today you eat plantain, and tomorrow you eat plantain, and the day after tomorrow you eat plantain, and every day for five years you eat plantain. Isn't it normal that after a while you are going to want to eat yam?"

"Maybe," I offered. "But if it happens that my plantain gets replaced not by yam but by cassava, I'm going to be miserable for the next five years."

You Know about Satellite Phones?

Sunday, 13 July 1997

Must go up for evening rounds. The nurse on duty has been having a drinking problem lately—he goes through stages; we have been in this one many times before—and needs to know that I am looking over his shoulder. He's not a bad nurse. Short and squat, a preacher's son married to a tall muscular vivacious southern woman whose wrong side I would not like to be on, especially if I were Edouard's height. The other night he came to my house for something, but he was smashed, and once he got here he couldn't remember what he had come for, and as he reached the door I saw big Alice, the wife, rounding the corner into our courtyard. She hung back at first, and she was not smiling. When Edouard moved aside to try to recollect what it was he had come for, Alice marched forward and started pouring out her grievances for me, mincing no words. Edouard, pretending to be out of earshot (no one in Kolofata was out of earshot), stood off to the side, back to us. After Alice had said her piece and excused herself and marched off, Edouard came back toward me and mumbled incoherently something about his wife appearing to have a lack of confidence in him. Eventually he waddled off. They have three children: Sonny, Aristotle, and a one year old girl they named Prudence, which is also the name of the leading brand of condoms in Cameroun.

Tuesday, 15th July. Tuesday night and I am looking forward to going to bed and hoping I get to stay there until morning. We've been buffeted back and forth several times over the past 24 hours, and although just about everything has worked itself to a satisfactory conclusion, we are tired. Yesterday was Monday, complicated this week by the arrival of a woman evacuated from one of our health centers for term pregnancy [with] eclampsia. She had already convulsed once and gone into a brief coma, and her blood pressure on arrival was still climbing. We got her under control and returned to our crowd of more run-of-the-mill patients, but she kept us on our toes all afternoon and anxious all evening. In addition to her we had 4 or 5 other patients who were (are) struggling and who could at any moment take a disastrous turn for the worse. Nevertheless I went to bed, but was not there long before a knock at the door had us both up again. The message was that something had "exploded" at the hospital and there was no power now to 2 of the 3 buildings. Exploded? I asked, visions of gas bottles and 40-liter jerricans of diesel and gasoline. Exploded, I was assured. Up we drove, in a hurry. Relieved, on the one hand, to learn that there had been no explosion—rather a bit of a fizz in one light fixture before the circuit blew—we were nevertheless dismayed to find the place in darkness. Except, fortunately, for the ward and maternity, and therefore the room where our eclamptic patient lay. A quick look around revealed no obvious fault, so we only checked plugs and sockets and circuit breakers—nothing charred—and turned things off and fired up the gas fridges. We know of no reliable electrician between here and Yaoundé—they must exist, but the dozen or so we've been through have not happened to be among them.

So we pondered, as we stood outside the darkened OPD, what to do and decided we would go search out our local hack and tell him to check first thing in the morning to see if it might luckily be something not too complicated. This we did, and as we left him to drive the rest of the way home, there was a little popping sound under the steering wheel and all our lights went out. And I thought, really, the sorcerers are out in force tonight. It is scary to drive at night without lights in our village—people think nothing of sleeping in the roads. But we got home and went to bed and woke up in the morning and went up early to the hospital.

And now I can finish my tale of woe quickly. Our local hack had gone up in the middle of the night, discovered (he decided) that rainwater had got into an outdoor light fixture and shorted it, blowing a fuse. He dismantled this light, rigged the fuse with a strip of foil from a pack of cigarettes, and by the time we got there in the morning there was light. The fridges, microscope, everything was fine. The eclamptic was fully dilated and delivered without complication a healthy girl. She had a post-partum hemorrhage that sent our own blood pressures through the roof, but we got that [stopped] after a bit of scrambling and murmured prayers. And the Land Rover we sent to Mora with Bello, who brought it back within the hour, a snapped wire repaired.

In addition to our internal electrical problems, general power outages occurred with infuriating regularity, always worse during the rainy season, and always, seemingly, at the worst possible time. One Sunday evening in late September after work had officially ended for the day I still had a young man paralyzed from the waist down sitting in the chair in my consulting room, five toddlers with temperatures over 105 degrees lying on mats in the waiting room, and a newborn who had decided to stop breathing. I was working on him in the ward when a nurse came to tell me that a woman had just delivered in the delivery room and had a bad tear he did not think he could repair properly. It was at this moment that the lights went out. In chaotic situations I found the best tactic was usually to look after one thing and then move on and manage the next and then the next and the next, and this is what we did. We convinced the newborn to breathe again, the young man was seen and admitted, we got all five toddlers to defervesce, and by the light of an otoscope we repaired the perineal tear, snipping off the last bit of suture with particular satisfaction.

Friday, 12 September 1997

AA came up unexpectedly Wednesday, bringing with him this brand new satellite phone called Planet I, and he wanted at all costs to get it working so he could call Yaoundé. The instrument is American and all the instructions are in English. We had dinner, and [AA] informed me that he was going to put me to work that night with Boukar [his bodyguard] so that he could call Yaoundé. "You know about satellite phones?" he asked. "I've heard of them," I said. "Good. Then you can figure it out. Boukar is waiting for you. I must call tonight." And then I was called away to see a man who'd been shot in the arm and while at the hospital there was a woman in labor and the nurse on duty was drunk so I was delayed, and when I finally got back home it was 10 o'clock and Boukar was still waiting for me. We got the various parts spread out on a table and sorted the papers and booklets and read them through and then started going along step by step. It did not seem difficult, but we would [reach] a certain step and get stuck. I finally told Boukar we should take it up to the hospital, which is on a hill, and try there. And lo and behold. When the [machine] started beeping as it does when it finds a satellite, the two of us could not control our giggles. I asked him if he knew a number we could try, and he chose one from Yaoundé, where he lives. After dialing, a recorded voice came on saying the call could not be completed as dialed and either try again or get help by dialing 11. Boukar didn't understand any of this, as it was in English. He had thrust the receiver back at me when he heard the strange voice. I told him to hit 11. Again a strange voice, and again he thrust the receiver back at me. An American voice. Male. Crystal clear. Sounded like a movie star to me. Asking what number we were trying to call and telling us what we had done wrong and what we had to do to try again. Very kind, very polite. And there I was talking American, and Boukar was trying to control his giggles. Not that I could control mine. It was eleven o'clock at night, we were standing in the black night on a hill at the edge of a village at the end of the world talking American to a handsome movie star (I know he was handsome) who was God only knows where and who had known ("It shows here, Ma'am, that you dialed 101 instead of 00.") what we had dialed and I got to wondering whether he knew about the gunshot wound and the woman who had just delivered. Boukar redialed according to our new instructions and the call went right through. He spoke for only a minute and when he hung up I thought, what the heck. You haven't really tested the thing if you haven't tried to call across the ocean. So I did and it was fun and just wonderful to talk to you, even so briefly. After hanging up we dismantled the phone and packed it all back up again and scurried down the hill so AA could make his call. I told him I had called you—I assume he gets billed somehow—and all he did was smile and clap his hands. His call went through with no problem, and he was delighted.

Write Well to the Big People, Tell Them about This Place

KOLOFATA'S CLIMATE ALLOWED for the harvest of two millet crops a year: the rainy season crop and the dry season crop. The first was harvested in late October, the second in February.

The year 1997 was not a good one for the wet season millet. The rains had started well, but they stopped six weeks before they were supposed to stop, and as a result many villages had almost total crop failure. Stalks grew to a good height, but then, without water or clouds, everything baked in the sun. Heads of grain failed to form. Leaves turned yellow and then brown and then so brittle that the slightest touch reduced them to powder.

We spent one harvesttime Saturday driving through the northern half of our district, the half worst hit. Going from village to village we saw the same devastation everywhere. In a couple of villages several elders insisted on climbing into the back of the Land Rover and guiding us from field to field.

One chief kept pointing, out one window and then out the other, saying, "See? See? That is our millet, and that and that and that. All of it, the heat has eaten."

We drove on in silence, reached another field, and then he said again, "All of it, that and that and that. No water. The heat has eaten it all. See? See? There and there."

Normally at this time of year famers cut their millet, piled the stalks up in a field, and left them for several days to dry. Teams of men wielding cudgels that looked like thick hockey sticks then pounded the heavy heads, loosening the grain. Usually it took several men two or three days to beat the millet off the stalks and bag the grain. A decent field produced enough to fill dozens of huge burlap sacks.

In one village we came upon a group of men pounding a pitiful pile of harvested heads. The amount of grain that would be reaped for the entire village could not fill one sack. A woman who had carried water to the field for the men to drink came over to the Land Rover.

"This year the millet did not come," she explained. The violet veil covering her head was frayed at the edges, and her *pagne* was faded to a faint yellow. I noticed the thinness of the soles of her flip-flops. "What are we going to do? What are we going to eat?"

At yet another village we got out of the vehicle and walked among the desiccated stalks. An elder approached.

"Please," he said. "You can help. Write well to the Big People in the capital. Write very well. Tell them that in this place the heat has eaten all the millet."

In fact a week earlier we had talked to Amadou Ali about what we had heard about this part of the district. He had indicated that there might be hope for some relief, and this was why we had decided to come see for ourselves.

We broke off a couple of withered, powdery unopened heads of grain, and after returning to Kolofata we boxed them up and sent them to Ali along with a report of what we had seen. We knew that if anything could be done, he would do it.

The price of millet tripled that year, reaching just over 30,000 CFA a sack. But aid came in time to the areas hardest hit, and no one in our district died of starvation.

Monday, 23 Mar. 1998.

I was called last night for what turned out to be [a] case of meningitis. We are up to 24 for the district so far, and it will go much higher. Today 74 medical consultations, another 20 antenatal consultations, 50 or so babies for vaccinations, 25 eye consultations in addition to 4 [eye]surgeries, 10 new hospital admissions, 3 women miscarrying, 1 staff meeting, and then we came home. And as I jumped down from the Land Rover, there came Bello walking across the lot with an envelope in his hand which I knew was from you. Very nice.

Everyone continues to do well, including the meningitis from last night. And the young man with tetanus; and the man with TB who had been down to 60 pounds; and the other meningitis patient who had been in coma; and the boy who had swilled some kerosene, vomited and aspirated the stuff into his lungs; and all three seriously dehydrated babies; and the teenager with heart failure caused by anemia caused by we're not yet sure what; and the other teenager who came in on the weekend with a seven centimeter gash through the tissues, muscle included, of his right thigh. "Fell on a bottle," he said, but I doubt it. He belongs to a tribe whose boys start wearing—and using—knives not long after they learn to walk without falling, and they are forever getting into fights and coming in with spectacular wounds. They hate scuffles with the law and will often invent stories to explain these lacerations. Either that or it is astounding how prone the male members of that tribe are to falling on bottles, running into trees, and having bizarre encounters with bicycle spokes, bridles and farming tools. He's doing fine, in spite of having lost a good deal of blood. Wanted to know this morning if we'd be taking the sutures out today. No, I said, you're with us till Saturday. He groaned: till Saturday! As if Saturday were longer than forever.

Whatever You Do, Don't Say You're from English

Sunday, 10 May 1998

We continue to—just what is the word? Sizzle does not do justice to the pressure one feels, as if the heat is actually pushing up against you. Swelter is heavier, but not quite hot enough. Burn is hot, but unmuggy. Suffocate conveys the sense you have that it is not really air that you're breathing but rather heat, molecules of air that have been transformed into molecules of heat that go into your lungs and diffuse into your blood so that the hot—sizzling, sweltering, burning, whatever—comes not just from the outside in but from the inside out as well. The body trapped in the middle, uncomfortably. Everyone says that this is the hottest hot season in memory, and I am certainly among those who believe it.

In Kolofata, tempers became fragile in the heat and patience wore thin. There were times when by the end of the day I was practically bouncing in my chair from the effort required to tug answers out of patients. This time of year by mid-afternoon it was 115 degrees in the room, and the ceiling fan, creaking gently through its whir, could only swirl all that warm air around, yet turning it off was out of the question. I kept the windows of my consulting room closed, since the air outside was even hotter, but the ultrafine sand being blown about during those months leading up to the rains still seeped through the cracks and plastered the wet back of my neck and my wet arms and the sweat-moistened desk and paper on which I was trying to write. Only by slapping the paper with a rag could I make the ultrafine sand scatter enough so I could jot another line or maybe two.

One May afternoon I was fighting this battle. We were supposed to be closing up in an hour, but there were still two benches of people waiting outside my door, and in the maternity a woman miscarrying would have to be seen, and in the ward a snake-bitten boy had just started bleeding again. I had seen forty-three patients since morning. Number forty-four walked into the consulting room and sat down.

She was a woman in her midfifties, and she looked well. I took her carnet, the small booklet in which we recorded hospital visits, and I asked her name.

"Falta Boukar," she said.

"Falta Boukar?" I asked. I looked carefully at the cover of the carnet and leafed through its pages and said, "Here it says 'Amina Modou.' This is the carnet of Amina Modou."

Unfazed, the woman craned her neck to look over at the carnet as if she could read, which she could not, and she replied, "Yes, yes, same thing," and then she launched into an explanation of why she had two names.

In fact I knew too well that people in Kolofata often had two or three or four completely different names, and as the explanations tended to be lengthy and I was tired and hot, I cut her off and took her word for it.

She accepted this, settled down, and adjusted the gold-flecked red veil on her head.

"Where are you from, Falta?" I ventured, and Falta pointed emphatically to the west and said decidedly, "France."

I scrutinized her, knew she had been coached. Because of the two countries' histories and subsequent ties with European powers, Nigerians and Cameroonians not uncommonly called their countries English and France. This woman was from Nigeria, surely, and since Nigerians paid slightly higher fees than Cameroonians, someone had told her to avoid telling us she was from English but rather to insist she was from France.

So she sat in her chair and repeated that she was from France. Usually patients were coached better than that. They would choose one of the dozens of villages that straddled the border and say, for example, Kerawa France or Limani France or Assigassia France. When I pushed her for a village, she continued to say only "France." I wrote "Nigeria" on her carnet.

"What is the problem today?" I forged on.

She looked surprised that I hadn't noticed and after a moment's hesitation held her forearms out and flipped them over and back again. "I have no blood. Look," she instructed, implying that nothing could be more obvious.

I looked. Her forearms were perfectly normal. Her nail beds, her palms, her eyes—all were normal. "How long have you had this problem?" I asked.

"Fifteen," she replied, and she brought together the tips of all five fingers of her left hand and the tips of all five fingers of her right hand, and these she tapped together, right against left, once: ten. Then, the fingertips still together, she gave a little shake to the right hand alone: five.

"Yes," I said, "I understand fifteen. But fifteen what? Fifteen days? Fifteen weeks? Fifteen years?"

She nodded, readjusting the red veil, and said, "Yes. Exactly. Just so. That is it, aha!"

Moments like this were when the bouncing began. Getting upset would only prolong the misery; keeping calm was of paramount importance. So I just slapped the rag against the paper with a little more smack than perhaps was needed, and with patience and perseverance I eventually got to the bottom of what the problem really was and determined that we could do something to help her. Bouncing and slapping I finished writing her carnet and she took it and went off merrily. Number forty-four out, number forty-five in.

Wed., 18 May 1998

What on earth is going on with Bill Clinton? I have been reading some newspapers and magazines I picked up in Maroua last week, and we seem to be the laughing stock of the world. But Hillary a hero, at least in the African press which contends predictably that a woman ought to show a decent tolerance for the dalliances of her man. No African I have spoken with comes even close to fathoming—and the higher up they are the further they are from grasping—how a common citizen, to say nothing of the female variety, can be such a thorn in the side of the most powerful man in the world. Back when this latest crisis started, someone asked me why we were so reluctant to let our presidents have affairs. I told him that whatever the reason for that, the real problem had more to do with lying than with having affairs. The nuance is grasped by few, and I found it in not one of the jeering articles I read.

Of the Pain They Bear, How Much Is Our Share?

Wednesday, 9 December 1998

Midnight, but [I can't] sleep. . . . We received a woman this afternoon from one of our health centers. Seven months pregnant, with two small children at home. Presented this morning with the complaint that her belly was getting bigger and bigger by the minute since last night. The nurse at the health center recognized something bizarre going on and brought her right in. The poor woman was conscious, feverish, covered with sweat, and her abdomen was hugely distended with air. After an initial assessment we took her to ultrasound and watched the fetal heart beating its last and saw the gas in the uterus and outside in the abdominal cavity, everywhere, some horrible gas-producing bacteria running rampant inside her. Surgery was not an option, and even if it were it could hardly have made any difference. We loaded her up with antibiotics. A gesture. When I left the hospital hours later, she was still alive, still covered with sweat, staring out of trapped-animal eyes, every breath an effort because of the mass of her abdomen pressing up against the diaphragm. Even around the IV site in her hand gas bubbled under the skin. Here she was this young woman, her living done, her children left behind, her days ending in this hideous fashion, and she was alert, aware. Life waning before her eyes, before our eyes, and even to comfort her I could do nothing.

Earlier in the day an eight year old sickler, a girl, came in crisis. Her cousin, a boy, is already on bed with us receiving treatment for an osteomyelitis in his leg. He is a couple years older—quite old for a sickler in these parts to still be alive. He fractured his femur last year and was treated in his village by the local bonesetter and the infection stems from that. We have known him since we came here and have cared for him from crisis to crisis. Most of his life has been lived in the kind of pain few of us can imagine. We have also known his cousin, the girl who came today, since she was a baby. She, too, has gone from crisis to crisis and came in today bottomed out. No blood. Every breath an effort that demanded all her concentration and determination. Her father matched and as we got the transfusion going I watched her thin chest—covered with scars where over the years the local healers had made their nicks in an effort time and time again to get the sickness out—wondering whether it would keep going in and out, would she keep making that effort long enough for her father's blood cells to deliver the oxygen her heart so desperately craved. You root hard for these kids and you stand in awe of them, wondering how they do it, how they hang in there, wondering why they must bear so much pain, imagining that they—like Christ?—must be bearing some of your share for you. She hung in there. This afternoon she was sitting up on the side of her bed, legs dangling, exchanging shy giggles with her cousin across the way. She'll be okay I think. Until the next time.

Sunday, 20th Dec. How can it be eleven days later already? What a blur. Our [medical] students have been here, hanging on to the edge of everything, and I worry as usual that they are not getting as much as they could or should or hoped to get out of the elective because of my being pulled in ten directions at once—always, it seems, away from the center. The painters have been painting away—they are no trouble, though the place remains a mess and smells of toxic fumes—and the electrician from Maroua came, a prima donna, made a fiasco of the lights in the new building, had a temper tantrum when I told him I wanted to verify his work before paying him, and after stomping up and down heaved himself into his pickup and sped off and I consider myself lucky to have escaped his wrath unflattened. The lights still do not work so we have a little problem there to solve.

Wednesday, 17 February 1999

Starting a letter will keep me from falling asleep, which I am sorely tempted to do but I know that I would only feel worse for giving in. I am in Maroua. This is our third back-and-forth [trip] in five days and after arriving home after dark last night I was up much of the night transfusing a six year old boy, and then up again at 4:15 to get in rounds before having to hit the road once more.

So far the [two-week long] seminar has been an almost total waste of time, poorly prepared and sloppily presented, but it is making several people a nice wad of cash (thank you Care International) and giving others in charge of a project steps to check off and stuff on which to base a jargon-filled report which will be written and bound between shiny plastic covers, a plastic spiral in some primary color running down the spine. Which will then be skimmed dutifully by a few desk-bound people who are serious about Doing Something for the Third World. Then filed away and never looked at again. And all we will have to show for it—except for the handful of people who made the wad—will be a few deaths here, a few deaths there, a little more misery, a little more neglect, because all the doctors and a good chunk of the health professionals in a whole region were yanked away from their posts.

When we arrived at the conference site yesterday morning we found a crowd of people gathered around a doctor's car furiously shoveling handfuls of sand onto the engine. It was on fire. They had been looking for an extinguisher but to no avail. We carry an extinguisher in each of our cars and this was the first time we have had occasion to use one. It worked, too. The fire, which had resisted all that sand, went out immediately. The problem was a fuel line that had come loose and spilled fuel which was ignited by a spark. I felt Providence at work—here we are zipping back and forth between Kolofata and Maroua and we still manage to be in the right place at the right time: in the morning to put out a fire and in the middle of the night to save the life of a comatose child. One manages, in the midst of the fatigue and frustration, to feel a certain satisfaction.

Thursday, 04 March 1999

Tomorrow a team [will be] coming from Maroua to inspect the hospital and assess our shortcomings. I saw—from the side—the 50 page questionnaire they want to go over. The head guy on this team came alone a couple of weeks ago, unannounced, hoping he would grab me for a couple of hours. He had come in the back door of my consulting room, files cradled in his arm. Ho ho, I thought. I took him out the front door of the consulting room, the one that opens on the waiting room, and slowly and silently led him through the crowd—it was a Monday, and you had to be careful not to step on toes—and around through the alcove into which the crowd had overflowed and on out onto the verandah where it continued. Then I stopped and looked at him and smiled. He looked like he wanted to run. Which more or less he did. I offered him a few choices. We could ask all these people to wait. We could see if Myra could get free to help him. He could wait. No no no to all that. He would leave, he said, he really couldn't stay. What day, he said, would be a good day? I laughed. He didn't understand. No day is a good day, I assured him. But if we could know a week or so in advance I could arrange the schedule so that at least a nurse consultant would be on duty so I could be free. Yes yes yes, he said and he was already inching his way towards his pickup.

Sunday, 7 March. Tipped off that something was amiss at one of our health centers, Myra and I made a surprise visit and inspection there Friday afternoon. I went hoping that the rumors were only that, and suspecting that they were at least mostly that, and came back despairing. A rip-roaring black market is thriving there, every one of the nurses in it thick and the local community health committee (which was formed for the purpose of preventing such shenanigans) is right there in cahoots with the nurses. There are stashes of dubious drugs locked away in cupboards and drawers in every room. These are sold to unsuspecting patients, who imagine they are getting real treatment, and money taken under the counter goes directly into the nurses' and committee members' pockets. The health center pharmacy—which sells legitimate drugs and should earn the income necessary to restock its shelves and keep the health center functioning—is therefore being sabotaged by its own staff. The staff have a vested interest in seeing the pharmacy fail since once the pharmacy can no longer restock its shelves, the nurses claim it is only for the good of the population that they go to the market in Nigeria, buy up a stock of "drugs" and sell these to the sick.

Although many of our nurses were—had always been and would remain—a disappointment, a few were excellent. Given the paucity of physicians and other highly trained staff, they were required to master skills normally reserved for much more qualified personnel. Nurses with two or three years' training often played the role of doctor. Ward aides performed as nurses. Others with even less education sometimes stepped in to fill big gaps.

Iza was one of these. Short and slight of build, she glided more than walked. Her face in repose was a smile, and when she was thrilled or happy or amused, that smile exploded like a Roman candle. Dark parallel lines scarified her Kanuri cheeks.

In 1978 she had been one of the first people and the only woman recruited by the government to provide health care for the people of Kolofata. At the time of her recruitment she was twelve years old and had a fourth-grade education. The state required a new recruit to be at least sixteen, so Iza's father told the recruiter that his daughter was sixteen, and that was that.

In her role as *matrône*, she was a liaison between village women and healthcare staff. Mostly, she translated patients' Kanuri and Mandara into the nurses' French and then back again. With time, just by watching, she learned to inject and vaccinate, to examine pregnant women and deliver babies, to place perfusions and transfusions, to dress wounds and insert urinary catheters—in short, to do nearly everything that a fully qualified nurse might do.

Because of the generally poor quality of teaching and the shortage of resources, a fourth-grade education in a place like Kolofata was only just better than none at all. Iza spelled all words phonetically and scrawled, in large, rickety, roundish letters, two or three words per line. She wrote things like *a couché* instead of *accouché* and *les maternel* instead of *lait maternel*, and deciphering her patient notes could be a challenge. Dates expressed as numbers confused her. August 6 could be set down as *006/08* or *006008/* or just *086*.

Because she had been employed for so long, she had money. She owned her own house and went through a succession of husbands. Occasionally these men disputed the paternity of one or other of her five children, none of whom she chose to send to school. When one of her daughters-in-law died, Iza inherited a grandson whom she raised from infancy.

She knew everyone in Kolofata and most people in most of our villages. Her brain mastered an intricate web of demographic connections. She knew whose brother a niece of a cousin had married, and when. She knew how many children a great-uncle's wife had had, and where they all were and what they all did. She knew who was having a spat with whom over land or cattle or inheritance. She knew the leaves and branches of family trees going back multiple generations.

In the hospital the trained nurses were embarrassed by her, that she with her rudimentary education should be in a white coat no different from their own. But because of her facility with languages and her connections with the community, they needed her. Patients trusted her and told her their secrets, which she kept.

Iza's father's name was Madi, but everyone called him Chetima, the honorific for "Chief." He was chief not of a place like other chiefs but rather of a people—musical people, people who blew into pipes and beat tom-toms and danced and sang for crowds on special occasions: *les griots*. Some towns had three or four groups of *griots*; others had none at all. They were itinerant and traveled from village to village, and at times from country to country, animating at weddings, national and religious holiday celebrations, political rallies, and sometimes for no reason at all, just for the coins.

For organized events, an envelope was prepared in advance, but players stood to earn much more from individual spectators who would stride forward from the crowd during a song and flamboyantly slap a 500- or 1,000-franc note on the forehead of a performer. An enterprising band knew how to sprinkle songs with the names of wealthy listeners, flattering and praising them until each one in turn duly showed his appreciation.

At the end of the day all the money collected was given to the chief of the *griots*, and he would divvy it up among his people according to seniority, performance, and need.

Iza was Chetima's firstborn, and she had a younger brother and sister. After his death Chetima's chieftaincy would normally pass to his son. The father, however, recognized that Iza was a striver with pluck, while the boy was weak and disinclined to hard work, and so on his deathbed Chetima made it clear to other leaders and the canton chief that he wanted Iza to succeed him.

There was consternation and discontent over this decision when Chetima died, for women were not and could not be chiefs, but Iza stood her ground. Insisting that her father's will be done, she donned his sky-blue robes and gathered her troops—grizzled men, young bucks, and nasal-voiced singing ladies—around her. She accompanied them to as many performances as her hospital work schedule allowed. She cooked for them when they came into town. She listened to their personal problems and tried to help when she could. She was fair in her distribution of the earnings. She was a good chief.

Tuesday, 30 March 1999

11 P.M. Just down from the hospital where a one year old fit beautiful chubby boy named Ali Mohamed is dying of croup, which crept in in the aftermath of measles. He lies cradled in his grandmother's arms, his jaw dropping with every intake of breath, the air scraping against raw swollen airways as it goes down, and you can tell by the way the chest strains hungrily that the oxygen is not getting down all the way. The mother crouches beside, struggling with panic, hope, disbelief. Watching the heaving chest, the dropping jaw, the closed eyes. Is it lack of blood? she asks. No, I say, it is the throat, the chest. She takes a tiny foot in her fist, then a hand. Still warm, still hope. Again I put a stethoscope to his lungs and her frightened eyes implore me to tell her he will be okay. But he will not. He is tired of trying, and there is nothing we can do but wait. I hate measles. It is a vicious bully of a disease.

The feast day [Tabaski] fell on Sunday and AA once again had a fine ram delivered to our door. It was prayed over and subsequently slaughtered with due ceremony then butchered, packed into a big carton and carted up to be distributed among our many patients unlucky (or lucky?) enough to be spending the holiday in hospital. We were recipients of whole meals carried over in covered pots on metal platters.

Holy Saturday, 3 April. Yesterday was Good Friday, the public holiday for Easter. With minimal staff on duty we were kept busy from our first case at 7:30 (urinary retention necessitating catheterization through an aging prostate) to our last at midnight (a criminally induced abortion, botched).

Apart from the run-of-the-mill pneumonias and measles, we had weird cases, some sad, some eerie, as if they had been saved up specially for Good Friday. A young mother with pneumonia on top of what I think is going to turn out to be leukemia. A three month old with hydrocephalus. A four year old with kidney failure. A fifty year old burned out leper, a woman who collapsed and then started acting strangely a day after a cooking pot fell off a hangar roof onto her head. Two cases of tetanus, a two year old boy and a three year old girl. It's been a long time since we've seen tetanus and then two arrive at the same time. Both from Nigeria. I don't know how many patients we saw, but we hospitalized 15 of them. The hospital [has] bodies everywhere inside and out. One tiptoes gingerly to avoid inflicting pain.

And another bizarre case yesterday. An old man—"old" is fiftyish, but his life had run its course—died of TB out under our trees where his family had dumped him several weeks before. A Christian family who apparently were mad at the old guy for having run off to Nigeria ten years ago and converted to Islam before limping back last month tubercular and in need of help. They brought him to hospital but refused to pay for his treatment, just left him there with a young daughter or daughter-in-law who stayed for a while but then took off as well, leaving him alone under the trees. We started treating him for free, which is against policy in cases where the family is not destitute, as his was not, but it was too little too late. I don't know who was feeding him. Maybe finally no one. Nor did I think he was that close to death. But this morning his body was there, curled up as usual under his favorite tree, but no longer breathing, and cold as the night sand. Men materialized this afternoon to wrap him in white cloth, bundle him into a cart and carry him off to be buried in the Muslim graveyard. I couldn't help but wonder where all these men were when he needed them.

Easter Sunday. You will be writing to tell me how beautiful the Mass was last night, and I can only tell you that it is during Holy Week and Easter that I most miss having church. Our work is our church, and the Passion is every day, the dying and the rising. But I would like to see a lily, a candle on an altar. I would like to hear a brass bell ring out with surprise and exuberance, a bit of Glory to God, an alleluia or two.

Thank you for your letters—they are the wind at my back.

~~~

The *Sous-Préfet* Wants to See You

Sunday, 11 April 1999

[Friday] a first-time pregnant woman came in from somewhere well beyond our District, in labor three days, dead baby stuck inside. Unable to urinate because the baby's head pressed up against the urethra, squeezing it shut. Urinary catheter wouldn't pass. Tiny nasogastric tube wouldn't pass. Bladder filled to her umbilicus. We ended up tapping it, to her great relief, but even with an empty bladder her efforts to push did nothing. So we hooked up the vacuum and with much pumping and straining and sweating got the baby out. I guess she'd sensed he was dead because when he came out she did not glance over, she asked nothing, she just held out her hands, a huge smile on her face, and said thank you thank you thank you.

Then the sous-préfet *summoned me. The* sous-préfet *is the government's Man on the Spot. Our U.S. system has no equivalent, but he is the official authority figure in the area. A southerner, he knows nothing about anything locally and except for the requisite kowtowing, the people pay him no heed. But he is feared. He can (or it is believed he can) have you hauled in, interrogated, tortured, locked up, deported. . . . He has the right to wear a military type uniform (the sleeves just a little too short, the jacket not quite matching the pants, the seat with that shiny over-ironed look, the cap fraying at the edges, the gold barred* epaulets flapping at one end) which this particular one does not do except on national holidays. This is the fourth sous-préfet we've been through since I've been here: they do not last long, and the first half of their stay tends to be dominated by rituals related to their coming, and the second half of their stay tends to be dominated by rituals of their going. Otherwise they have little to do except pester people, and some of the people they particularly like to pester are those in charge of the public services in their area. Including health. Ta-da. The typical thing is, I'm in the middle of a 60 patient day, an old man has just fainted on the back verandah, a toddler is convulsing in the waiting room, the nurse in the delivery room is calling me, a supplier is delivering a carful of office supplies, and a messenger pops in to tell me, "The sous-préfet wants to see you." I [remove] my stethoscope and jacket and take off in the Land Rover as the roomful of sick people in the waiting room follow me with their eyes and I can feel their despair. I get up to the sous-préfecture and knock and walk into his office, the cold of the air conditioner blasting me, and there he is sitting back in his big padded chair behind his big empty desk reading a novel or a newspaper or talking to a relative on the phone (his is the only phone in town). We greet and he asks me to sit down and he wants to talk about the weather or about a sick relative or about a meeting or about some report I sent him or something. A couple of times he asks me how the hospital is and I tell him we are really busy and I do the necessary amount of [checking] my watch when it looks like he's forgetting that I've other people to tend to. All the time I am searching for the moment to stand up and make it look like it was his idea that I do so.

Friday. Let's see—Friday we had just finished the vacuum delivery and an 18 year old boy who had come Wednesday in coma had just died and an old man had just been dumped outside my back door and was moaning in pain, I did not yet know from what, and a one year old so dehydrated you could see the space between his eyeball and his socket was outside my other door—when the messenger came. "The sous-préfet wants to see you." I got the one year old started on treatment, made sure the old man wasn't dying, took off my stethoscope, got into the LR. Fifty patients' eyes following me forlornly, and [I] thinking bitterly, How can you leave them like that? But I do. Up to the sous-préfecture. Knock knock. Blast of cold air. He's snug in his padded chair—headrest, padded armrests—fiddling with a radio. "Can't get Yaoundé," he explains helpfully. "Ah," I say, nodding. We greet, I sit. How's the hospital? he says. Busy, I say. Wants to know how the measles epidemic is. I tell him. Meningitis? No epidemic yet, I tell him. He is glad. Asks me to write up a report, in case anyone calls and asks him. Be happy to, I tell him. Talks about the weather, about who he's thinking of calling to service the air conditioner. Mentions that I left the meeting early last Thursday. A meeting at the sous-préfecture this was. I'd come to the hospital an hour early—6:20—to get a jump on seeing patients that day, knowing I had a meeting. Yes, I tell him, but the meeting was called for 10:00 and I was there at 10:00 and it didn't get started for another 45 minutes, and really there's only so much time I can cut out of a day. He apologized for starting late, it had nothing to do with him. It was his meeting, but "No no," I said, "of course not." So it went and so it went, until I seized that moment which appeared to be opportune for standing up.

Our snakebite [patient from] last weekend is a traditional healer—a col-
league, as I keep telling my staff, to their displeasure. On the day he came he had
no money to pay for treatment (about $26—antivenom is expensive) so we took
his satchel of barks and roots as collateral. Relatives came up with the money the
next day. He has had a steady stream of fellow healers—each with his leather
sack slung over his shoulder—coming to see him, which I have enjoyed.

At the end of April the new préfet of Mora went on his introductory tour of
the towns and villages of our *département*, the administrative division to which
Kolofata belonged. Every time a new préfet was appointed, a new tour took place,
and as the health authority in Kolofata and head of the public hospital, I was
obliged to join the touring group. These tours were ghastly affairs. Lasting several days and usually sprawling across weekends, they consisted of endless hours
spent in the searing heat and choking dust listening to the same speech over and
over again. My morning rounds at tour time had to be done well before dawn,
and my afternoon rounds well after dusk, so for me such days were always very
long and very tiring.

Usually the messages the préfet came to impart were laudable, and in an illiterate setting where communication is mostly by word of mouth, the government
had few other options at its disposal if it wanted to speak to the people.

This time there were nine points that the new government appointee
expounded upon at length at each stop: (1) Keep the peace. (2) Avoid dependence
on other countries—by which he meant Nigeria—for your economic well-being.
(3) Send your children to school. (4) Go to a health center when you are sick. (5)
Organize yourselves and undertake work in groups. (6) Don't be content to work
only during the three-month farming season; get up from under the trees and do
something productive. (7) Don't be waiting for handouts from other countries—
the food aid they send you is the fruit of their own labor, and they have surplus
because they work hard, not because their climate is any better than yours; in
fact it is worse. (8) Don't be asking the federal government for this and that and
the other thing until you've done something for yourselves first: build your own
school, fix your own road, organize your own grain reserves. (9) Stop cutting
down trees and refusing to replant. What exactly do you think your children are
going to do when you've used up all the firewood?

They were worthy messages, but I wondered if the pomp, smacking as it did of
old colonialist days, added to or detracted from the likelihood that they would be
heard and taken to heart. I resented being yanked away from my patients and felt
the entourage needed me as much for my Land Rover as for anything else. Nine
burly men, the heads of all the government services in the district, were stuffed
into the back of my sweltering Land Rover as we lumbered from village to village.
Surprisingly, the men didn't seem to mind being piloted by a skinny, old white

woman, and in fact they seemed to enjoy watching people in the villages wave and clap and shout as we drove by.

"Ha!" the men remarked at several of those villages. "It is the préfet's *tournée*, but you are the one they applaud!" And it was true, and that was not unenjoyable.

There Is a Huge Difference between 108 and 112 Degrees

Tuesday, 11 May 1999

Merry month of May, and we are sweltering. One sleeps bathed in sweat, hair matted to the back of the neck, waking up ten or fifteen times a night to get unstuck from the mattress, to shower, to drink, to shift, to break some strange dream. All day long you are thirsty and nothing is as sweet as a tall cold glass of water. A cottage industry has started at the hospital as women from civil servant families [with] fridges fill plastic bags with water—about 2 cups' worth—and tie them shut, store them in the fridge then in the morning pack them into a cooler and send a son up to sell them at the hospital for 7 cents apiece. We have so many patients and caretakers and assorted visitors these days, and it is so hot, and cold water tastes so good, they make a killing. Some women get fancy and fill a smaller plastic bag, mix in some colored sweet syrup, freeze these and sell them as popsicles—called "Alaskas" here.

Yesterday that hot dry desert wind swirled tirelessly all day long. It is like being followed at a couple of inches by a floor heater everywhere you go.

The wretched measles continues and our verandahs are still overrun. We lost a big boy—16 years old—last week, a terrible heartbreak. The mother had already lost a husband and two sons to measles in Mora, and she had come to Kolofata with four other sons. The eldest was in terrible shape and hung on and hung on but just never came round. One evening as I was doing rounds he called me over—no voice, just dry air coming through his swollen parched throat—and asked me for ice water to drink. I went out with my 7 cents and tried to find the boy with the bags of water in the cooler and I found him but he was sold out. I could have tried harder to get some cold water, but I got distracted and did nothing more, and two days later he was dead. And apart from feeling sad and angry at myself for having let him down—such a simple thing!—I can't help but wonder whether the outcome might have been different (it is absurd, and yet it's not) had he had that little taste of cold water, that little act of kindness.

Convincing parents to send their sons to school was difficult; convincing them to send their daughters was almost impossible. No one saw the need, and most adults believed that girls were incapable of school learning. Yet it was hard to see how health and economic development could advance if more than half the population remained illiterate and innumerate, particularly if most of that half was female. We hit upon an idea. Even if they could not get a formal education, girls could be taught to speak, understand, read, and write French, and if they could do that, then they would have a chance to interact more meaningfully with the world beyond their immediate communities. We proposed a ten-week course for girls aged eight to fourteen years old. An unused operating room would be converted temporarily into a classroom. With the help of civil servant wives and a local schoolteacher named Biye Mahamat, we would teach practical homemaking skills—things like cooking, baking, sewing, embroidery, and knitting—but we would do all the teaching in French, and a French language class would open and close each day. We presented the idea to parents, and a surprising number consented to send their girls.

> *Monday, 28 June 1999*
>
> *It is Monday morning, six thirty, and our girls' school is due to start this morning. Things are set up. We have cooking pots and firewood, knitting needles and yarn, cloth and thread, a foot pedal old-fashioned sewing machine, basins of flour, tubs of margarine, eggs, oil and whatnot. Forty-two girls signed up. I've contracted with a woman in town to provide 180 beignets a day for snack time. Each teacher has her objectives noted and we will see how it goes. I've reminded them that these are girls who, for example, have never seen a pair of scissors, let alone used them, and [who] speak no French, so it will be slow patient going. I will not be involved, as I have this other job, but I'll keep an eye on things from a distance.*

On the last day of classes for our girls' school, we invited parents to come see what their daughters had accomplished. In addition to the display of dresses they had sewn, napkins they had embroidered, and baby pants they had knitted, the girls gave readings and performed sketches, all in French. The parents, especially the fathers, were flabbergasted. "We had no idea," several of them said, "that our daughters could learn to speak like that." They promised they would no longer keep their girls at home when the school year started. Many of them honored that pledge, but for those who did not, we continued to offer the course every year until finally, many years later, the village had so few girls unable to speak French that we switched our focus to women. In the meantime, we moved the school out of the hospital and into a new building, a sort of women's community center, that we built down the hill from the hospital.

> *We had a rainstorm on Sunday. The farming season has begun. At the hospital we've dug holes and will be planting 500 saplings this weekend.*
>
> *We spent upwards of $600 repairing our various roofs (again, yes again) and the driving rain was altogether indifferent—came right through in more than a*

dozen places. At the end of the season we'll have to replace ceiling boards (again, yes again) and do some big-time painting repairs (again, yes again) and dream up our next scheme for keeping the water out next year. Much as the leaks drive me crazy, the patients are wonderful in their nonchalance. They are used to roofs that are so much worse (blown right off, for example) that they just shift their beds however they can to squeeze into a space between raindrops and waterfalls.

Wednesday, 11 August 1999

I've not written to a soul for over a week. Might as well be dead.

We were in Maroua for meetings last Thursday and Friday. On a scale of one to ten, ten being most useless, these meetings rated about a six hundred and thirty-five.

Sunday afternoon [I was called] to see a woman who had been evacuated from one of our health centers. In labor for four days, first pregnancy after a nine year struggle to conceive. Nigerian. Membranes had been ruptured for three days. Don't you wonder what they're doing all that time and how it can take them so long to clue in that getting help might not be a bad option? She was fully dilated but for a lip of cervix and the fetal heart had hung in there. The head was high, though not in the stars, and her pushes were getting her nowhere. We got out the vacuum. Myra usually provides the brawn needed to work the hand pump—a killer of a thing—but she had not come up, so I called our pharmacist and she came and tried her hand. And failed miserably. She's about my size, and that pump would have none of it. It demands altitude and upper arms of a certain diameter. Fortunately the nurse on duty was one of our taller more ponderous ones. I had thought I would need him to help pull the baby out, but I told him to have a go at the pump. He did and the pressure crept up and eventually, a faceful of sweat later, [he] got [it] to where it had to be. I tugged and guided the head, which glided along on our first try. The body followed easily, drenched in meconium. The nurse cut the cord (eyeful of blood as in my excitement I failed to blink on time and from now on I'm going to wear my glasses in the delivery room) and we resuscitated the little guy only a few minutes before he took over and proceeded on his own. And then never looked back. We put mother and baby on antibiotics and they've done fine, and the whole family thinks we're the best thing since fried plantain. Which, frankly, we are.

Thursday, 20 April 2000

As is usual for this time of year we are busy and could easily stay up there round the clock seeing patients. As soon as a patient enters my room I start thinking about getting him out—not a very healthy way of practicing medicine. You begin trying to diagnose them by the way they walk across the room, the timbre of their voice, the way the babies cry. Anything but straight answers drive me up the wall . . .

> *DR: Good morning, what is your name?*
> *PT (coughing, 55 year old grey-stubbled ramrod-straight villager, probably carried an antique rifle and half-filled someone's discarded army fatigues during the Biafra war): Meina!*

DR (writing): Meina?
PT: Blama Meina, suh!
DR (writing): Blama Meina?
PT: Present!
DR (looking at him, startled): Yes—good. What is the problem?
PT: I am coughing.
DR: Since when?
PT: My wife went to visit her sister.
DR: Yes but since when are you coughing?
PT: In Bama. Her husband—the sister's husband that is—died.
DR: That's when you started coughing?
PT: When would that be, suh?
DR (deep inspiration, controlled expiration): Blama Meina—
PT: Present!
DR: When did you start coughing?
PT: When did I start coughing?
DR: Yes, that's it!
PT: Two weeks ago.
DR (great relief, writing): Are you coughing up blood?
PT (bending over, rolling up a trouser leg): My knee hurts too—here.
DR (looking, reluctantly, at the knee, touching it, manipulating it, dismissing it as a fine normal knee): Did you injure it? Fall? Hit it?
PT: No no, all by itself it just started hurting. Swelled up like that.
DR (getting up, circling the knee, looking at it from all angles): It's not swollen. Where do you think it's swollen?
PT (peering down at the knee, squeezing it repeatedly with his fist): Oh well maybe not today.
DR: Blama, are you coughing up blood?
PT: What?
DR: Are you coughing up blood?
PT: Blood?
DR: Yes, blood!
PT: No—not much.
DR (glancing at watch, checking how many [patient] numbers are in the box, subtracting to figure out how many remain in the waiting room, calculating when, at this rate, the last one will finally walk through the door): Are you coughing up blood—any blood at all?
PT: Blood? No no—no blood.

And on and on and eventually somehow you get through the history and then there is the physical. ("Breathe deeply," you say, putting the stethoscope to his chest, and he inhales deeply—and holds it. You wiggle your stethoscope on his chest to get him to breathe out; he doesn't get it so you shake him gently and finally say, "Breathe out, breathe out!" and he does, and then you try to show him what you mean when you say "Breathe deeply," which is In and Out, and you do it, several items, wondering as you do if your patients when they do it feel as dizzy as you do when you do it. Many minutes later he finally has the knack of it so you can examine him and satisfy yourself that you have heard what you *think you have heard.) And you get to the end, and you watch him go and even more carefully watch the next patient enter, searching in the way he walks, the way he holds his head, the way his shoulders move, for any clue that might help to shorten this next encounter.*

The surgical building continues to look more and more like the real thing. We hold our breath for the usual two things that have given us such headaches in the past—does the electrician know what he is doing, and will the roof resist the rains?

Monday, 22 May 2000

I find there is a huge difference between 108 degrees and 112 degrees. With the former you notice that it is hot. With the latter you feel as though there are chains buckling all your muscles to the earth, as though your joints are fused, your pores clogged with sweat, salt, dust and grime. Oh May, such a lovely month in so many countries of the world, and this is not one of them.

Because of a close tally in Florida, demands for ballot recounts and legal proceedings that ultimately led to a Supreme Court decision to stop them, the results of the US presidential election held on November 7 would not be declared for another month, when George W. Bush would be pronounced victorious over Al Gore.

Sunday, 12 November 2000

I suppose that by the time this reaches you we will know who our next president will be—although not necessarily, from what I hear. We had Moussa turn on CNN Tuesday night and we remained transfixed for the next three nights. It is not an easy situation for non-Americans to understand and in Camerounians' minds, corruption must be at the core of it.

Sunday, 3 December 2000

The other day I crossed paths with yet another poisonous snake in nearly the same place I encountered one not long ago. I debated. I do not like killing snakes because I am not expert enough to kill them cleanly. They always end up writhing for a while and thrashing about and screaming soundlessly, their jaws open wide and their tongue thrusting and their eyes ablaze. You imagine them thinking, What did I ever do to you? So I don't like killing them. But then I thought, there are children around, and even if this guy can't help being what he is, his venom is just as venomous, so up—and then down—went my stick.

Saturday, 16th Dec. 2000

My last patient this morning was a guy of about 70 or 80 or 90 who sat in my chair and promptly held his left foot out to me. It was a dry scaly foot, of the kind that had walked through 70 or 80 or 90 hot seasons' worth of sand. A little swollen.

He recounted at length his tale of having been pierced by a thorn seven months ago just there at the base of the big toe. His foot had swollen to gigantic size, he said, oh you should have seen it, and finally one day when he could stand it no more his son took a razor blade and stabbed it and pus came gushing out, oh you should have seen it, and then, slowly, the foot got better. He sat back and watched me. I waited, watching him back, expectantly, but nothing else was forthcoming, so I asked, "Does your foot still hurt?" Oh no, no, no, he assured me, holding it out again for me to see. It is better. "Well, wonderful," I said. "So what brings you to the hospital today?" His full head of hair was cut short and trim and it was silvery white so he looked like he had just come in from a snowstorm, and his eyes were little and black and unblinking. I had a headache after that for a while, he went on to explain. This was hopeful—I got ready to write. You have a headache? I asked. No, no, he said, I did. For a while. I did have a headache for a while, but it got better. Now—he shook his head—no headache now. He wore charms on leather thongs around his biceps, across his chest, around his waist. A sheathed dagger dangled from a cord at the belt line. I ran through a few more symptoms—abdominal pains, urinary problems, cough, aching joints—and yes yes he had had all at one time or another. He seemed pleased to be able to tell me this. But no no, none of these things were troubling him just now. The man had spent a lot of money to come 50 miles for this consultation, and I spent fifteen minutes trying to figure out why, and, I might add, not succeeding. Since he started out with the foot story and since people here often think they can be poisoned either immediately or years down the line by walking on something put in their path by some enemy to poison them, I suspect he was coming to get checked out and antidoted against that. And I suspect he just figured I ought to know that, without him having to be so crass as to dot the i's. Anyway in the end he left pleased as punch with a month's supply of a couple of different colorful vitamins, and I believe or hope that these will do the trick.

I understand we managed to select a president-elect after all. Aren't we clever.

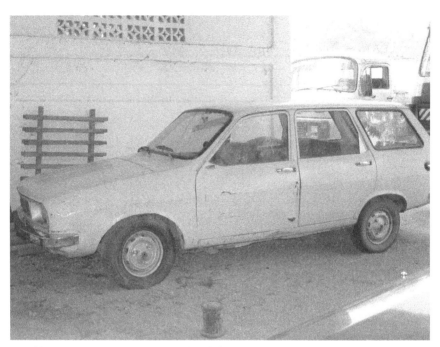

The old Renault 12, with stuck doors and little floor.

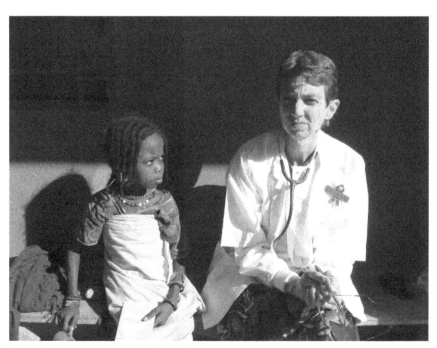

The author sharing a ray of sunshine with a young patient.

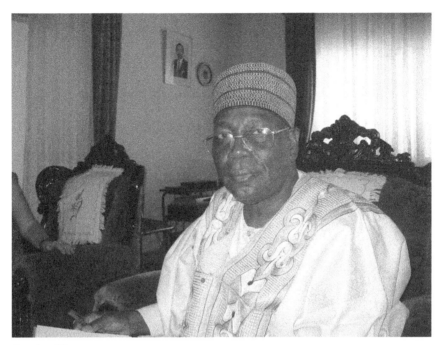

Amadou Ali.

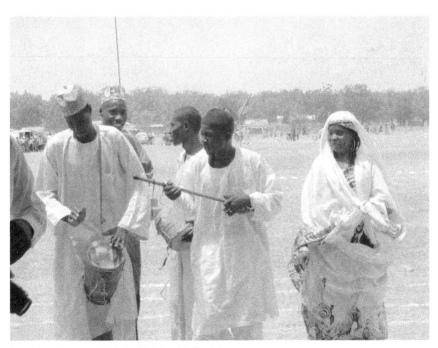

Local musicians, with their chief, Iza Madi, right.

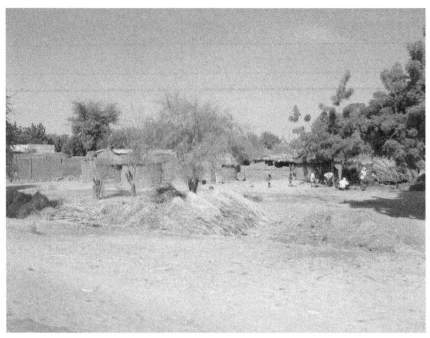

A village on the road to Kolofata.

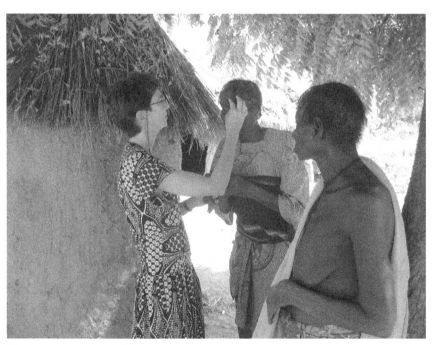

Checking a woman's painful eye.

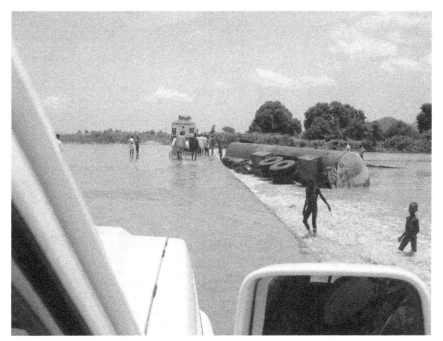

Oil tanker tipped off a flooded causeway.

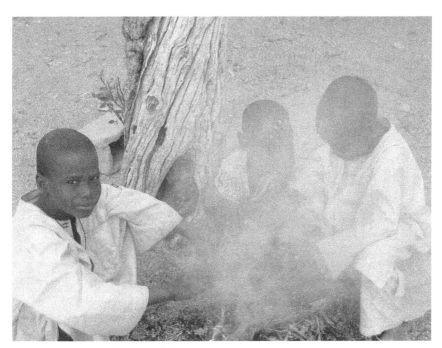

Boys warming themselves on a cold morning.

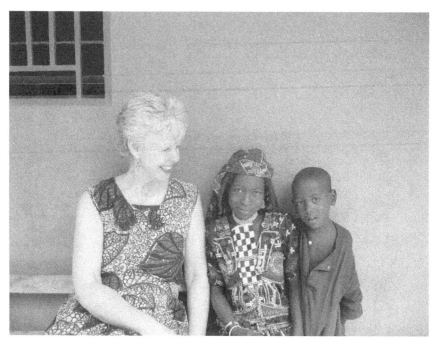

Myra with two young friends.

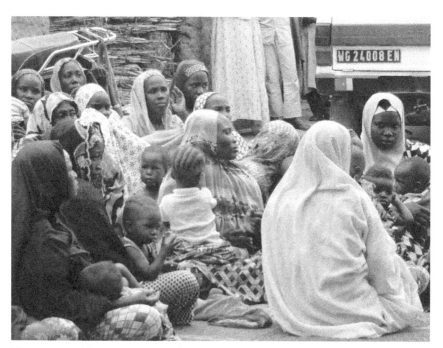

Women waiting for care at an outreach post.

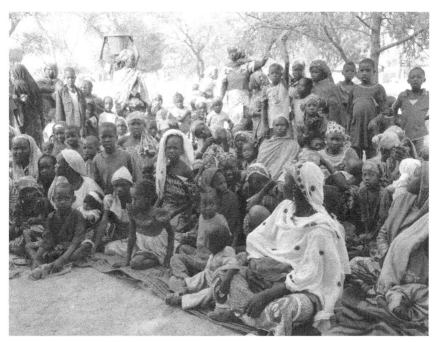
Townspeople assembled to hear a health talk.

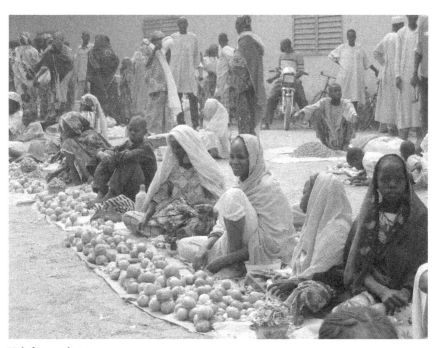
Kolofata market.

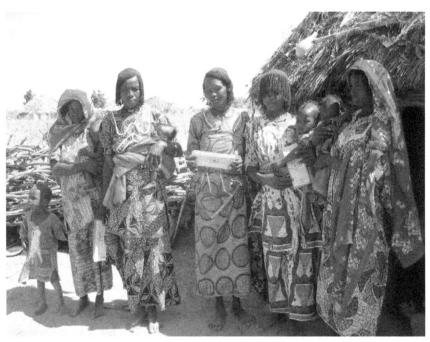

Women and children lined up for vaccination.

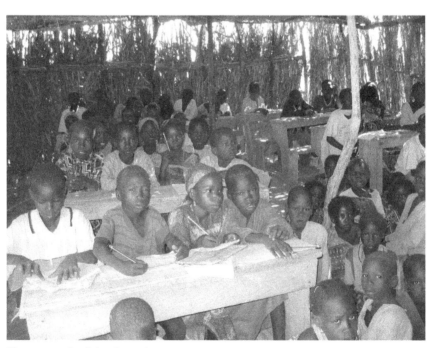

Elementary school class in session.

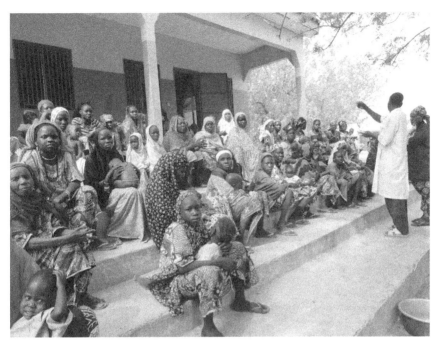
Women and children outside the pediatric ward.

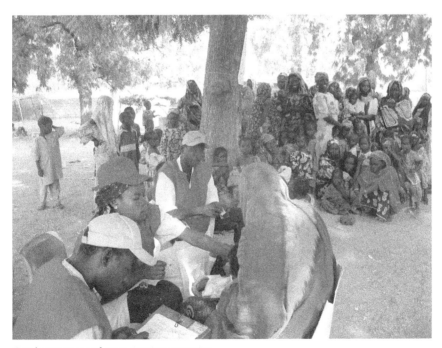
Conducting a measles vaccination campaign.

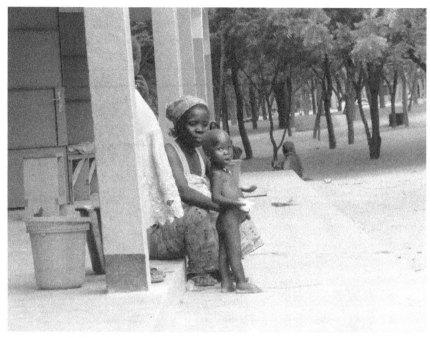

Woman and child on the hospital veranda.

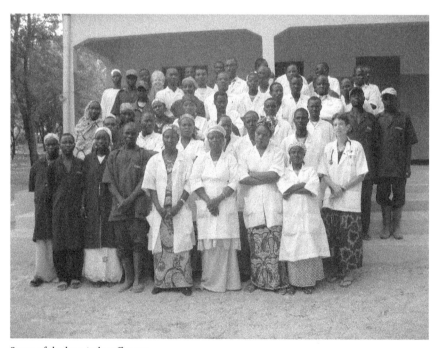

Some of the hospital staff, 2007.

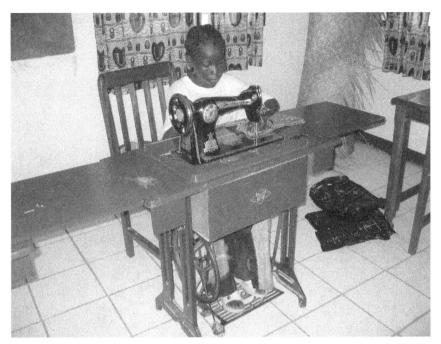

A girl learning to sew at the girls' school.

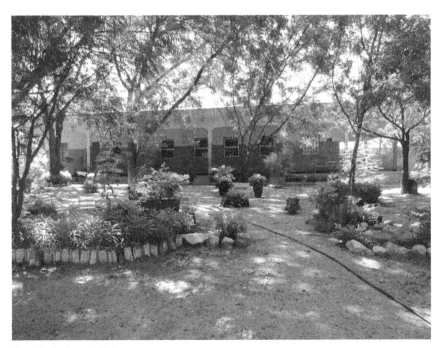

Outside the hospital lab.

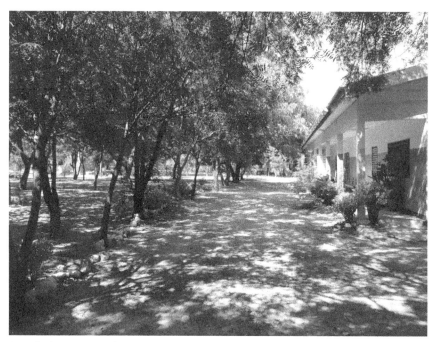

Outside the outpatient department.

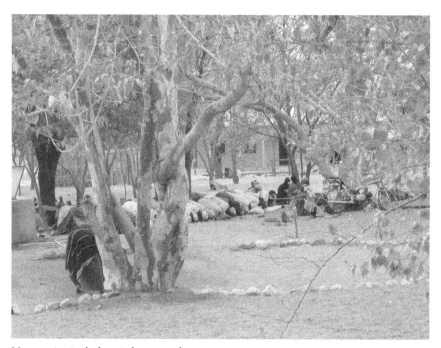

Men praying in the hospital courtyard.

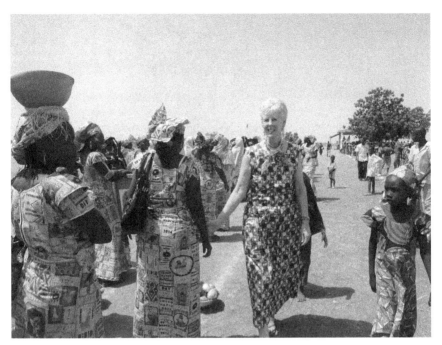

Myra greeting women on International Women's Day.

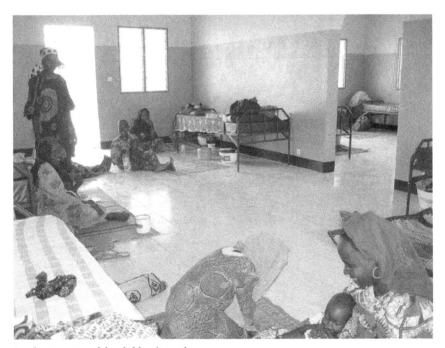

Inside one room of the children's ward.

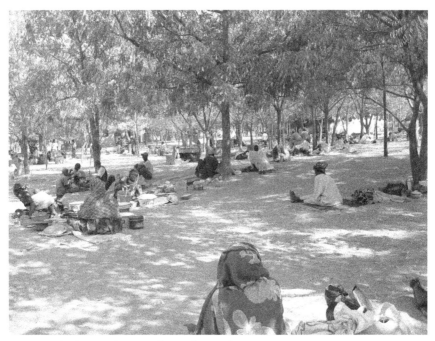

Patients and relatives relaxing on hospital grounds.

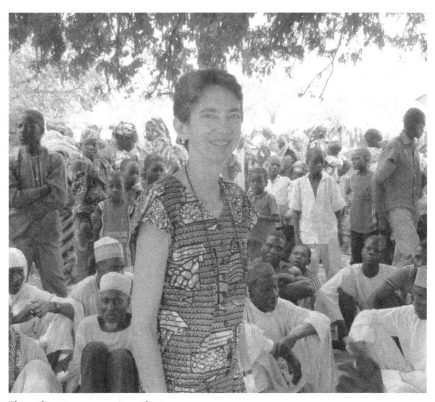

The author at a community gathering.

Part III

*Anyone who brings us regular power and water
will be president for life. It's that simple!*

Sekou Ahmed Cissokho, Guinean journalist

OUR PATIENTS WERE an unending source of inspiration. Their fortitude amazed me, their unadorned yet glittering verbal expressions kindled my imagination, and their perspectives, pragmatic and frank, constantly challenged my own.

Medically I was flying solo nearly all the time, and the frustration that came with being unable to discuss cases with other doctors, to compare notes with them or question decisions, never fully fell away. Yet to be confronted every week by cultural phenomena and by pathologies of a variety and magnitude few Western doctors would encounter in a lifetime was a unique and priceless gift. I knew how fortunate I was to have this, and I recognized repeatedly that there was no other work anywhere in the world that I would rather do or that I felt I could do better.

Their Ability to Cope Is Almost beyond Belief

Wed. 9th Jan. 2001

Yesterday, Madeleine [from our health committee] came to talk about AIDS. Here is part of what she said: "And you men. You sit out on the streets and you watch women walk by, and there is a woman with nice cloth and shoes, and clean, and she looks at you because she wants your money to buy some little things she needs. And so you take out your money and you go to this woman and

WITH YOUR VERY OWN MONEY you buy that sickness! Instead, you could have taken that money and gone home and given it to your wife so she could buy nice cloth and shoes and soap and then she would have been as beautiful and clean as that lady. But no." The men all nodded in agreement and swore to Allah they would never do such a thing again.

Not until 2005 did the government decentralize its HIV management program and make it possible for us to get medicines for treating patients with AIDS. In 2001 we were able to offer our AIDS victims little more than symptomatic relief.

Hadja, a twenty-five-year-old Nigerian woman who had both AIDS and tuberculosis, was one of these patients. Adama was her four-year-old daughter. Adama's father had already died of AIDS, and the rest of Hadja's family, ignorant and fearful of the disease, had dumped Hadja on our doorstep, evidently hoping never to see her again or risk being contaminated by her. Adama was deposited alongside her mother.

In Kolofata, as in most of rural Africa, patients' families looked after the feeding and nonmedical care of their hospitalized relatives. During her long hospitalization, no one came to visit Hadja, and so Adama was her mother's sole caretaker. She did all their laundry, swept the room twice a day, made porridge, carried water, collected firewood, went into town to buy things like matches and sugar, and emptied and cleaned her mother's bedpan. In the evenings they would sit together and chat, Adama telling her mother about things she had seen that day and at night they slept in each other's arms.

Adama was not quite expert at combing and braiding her hair, and she waged a running battle with lice. She had one flip-flop (not a pair) and one outfit—a blouse and a flimsy skirt—and on laundry day she would wash these, set them on the sand in the sun, and then crouch naked on the veranda waiting for them to dry. Her smile, which she was seldom without, was electric. She never walked if she could skip, never talked if she could sing, and all her songs, near as I could tell, she made up. She fashioned her own toys—dolls from bottles, finger puppets from wild mushrooms—and played with these and shared them with others, chortling with pleasure. The entire hospital staff were enthralled by her, and most of us were head over heels in love with her.

Slowly, as her TB was treated, Hadja's condition improved. She understood the nature of her illness and had told us she did not want to die in the hospital. Once she regained her ability to walk there was little reason to keep her confined. On a bittersweet morning we said our good-byes, Adama the proud new owner of a coloring book, a doll, a complete pair of flip-flops, and a few hand-me-down shirts given to her by one of our nurses.

Several months later, we received word that Hadja had passed away. I sent one of our health workers to their Nigerian village to offer the sympathy of our staff and to see how Adama was. The health worker returned late the same day and broke down in tears as she gave me report. She had found Adama huddled and crying alone in the hut where her mother had died. The family had confiscated Hadja's medicines; after leaving hospital, she had not taken another dose. Adama's doll, coloring book, new shirts, and shoes were gone. Adama herself had taken the clothes off her mother's dead body, washed them, and wrapped herself in them, for it was the rainy season and she was cold. Her uncle and his two wives refused to go near her.

It happened that in a distant Nigerian village there was an old woman and her old husband raising a six-year-old boy named Moussa who was said to be Adama's half brother. The old woman learned of Hadja's death and made the difficult journey to convey condolences to the family. Horrified by what she saw when she reached the compound and afraid that Adama would be sold into slavery, she offered to take the girl back with her. Adama's uncle gladly handed her over.

Eventually, the old woman managed to locate an aunt in yet another village, this one in Cameroon, and persuaded her to take custody of her young niece. One day I made my way to this village to see her.

As the Land Rover pulled up outside the aunt's house, Adama was peering from behind an open door. She charged toward me, face alight, and threw her arms around me. On her feet were plastic bags she had tied neatly with string at the ankles.

I chatted for a while with her and her aunt and uncle. After much coaxing they promised me they would send Adama to school. I realized it was a promise unlikely to be kept without a great deal more coaxing, so I made a mental note to hold him to it. As I got up to leave I handed Adama a few small gifts. One of these was a framed photograph of her with her mother, taken during their stay with us in Kolofata. Unaccustomed to looking at pictures, she studied it for some time before suddenly understanding what she was seeing. Then she jumped up, a giant smile lighting her face. She laughed and shouted with joy, "My mother!" and hugged the picture to her chest.

Tuesday, 14 August 2001

After a series of heavy rains six of our riverside villages succumbed to flooding. [Myra and I went to] the worst hit, and a good ¾ of it was leveled. We were greeted effusively by women and children, and everyone wanted to show us everything—the waist-high water line on what walls were left standing, the houses and kitchens and walls and stalls that had collapsed, the paths the rushing water had taken—it came from 3 directions at once—when it overflowed the banks of the rivers. But for the chipper women showing us around and the giggling bouncing crowd of children with upturned dirty but radiant faces following us everywhere, it would have been an unbearably eerie sight. Walls had turned back into mud, like a village of sand castles after the tide had come in and gone out. Straw roofs had survived to some extent, deformed and ragged conical things, [each one] incongruously large sitting on the ground like a snowman's hat in the spring. People had lost everything—clothes, money, food, pots and utensils, those little gold coins which are the essence of a woman's essential wealth, even (they hastened to tell me as if warning me not to be angry) even their health cards! (We kept them wrapped in plastic, one woman added, but it did no good.) All swept into the river. Most families had already cobbled together some sort of temporary shelter, using woven mats and millet stalks and recovered bits of metal sheeting—nothing even close to watertight, but shelter of a kind at least. Their resilience—their cheerful resilience—and ability to cope are almost beyond belief. It is the flip side, maybe, of their maddening acceptance of fate (as in "Why vaccinate my child—if God wants him to get measles, he will get measles") that we so blithely curse and wish we could turn around.

Sympathy and Shared Horror

FROM THE CRUSADES and the Spanish Inquisition to the Eastern European pogroms against the Jews and the rise of Islamic and Hindu extremism, religious fanaticism has helped define societies for hundreds of years. Modern Islamist extremism grew out of the partition of Palestine during the years following the Second World War, when flames of religious fervor were fanned as a means of adding heat to nationalist fires set to destroy the new state of Israel. All of that was far away, and even living in a predominantly Muslim community in Africa, I was no different from most Americans in thinking that Islamist extremism had nothing to do with me or my country. But as the summer of 2001 came to an end, things were about to change for all of us.

Saturday, 15 September 2001

We came home late on Tuesday and Moussa was waiting for me when I pulled into the compound. He had been at AA's watching TV. He had a look of distress on his face and blurted out, "Come. Something bad is happening chez vous." I thought he meant our house here—had something caught on fire? I wondered. "What?" I said, looking towards the house. "No," he said, "chez vous—over there," and he pointed up and over, as in up and over the sea. "Go put your things in the house and come." I didn't go put my things in the house, I followed him to AA's. The television was on and tuned to CNN and there it all was, the towers collapsing and the Pentagon burning and the planes crashing—2? 3? 4? 5?—and air traffic grounded and flights diverted to Canada and Bush sequestered and no one knowing whether whatever was happening was ending or beginning. It was confusing—had navigational systems been taken over? Air traffic control towers? Was some diabolical fiend sitting at some master computer somewhere? I stared in uncomprehending horror at the screen—as Americans and others all over the world must have been doing at that moment—and then suddenly, like a huge wave rolling in, the reality of what I was seeing hit me and I sat down and could not stop the flood of tears—of sadness and anger and fright. Only gradually did it become clearer—the hijacking, the suicides, the Pittsburgh crash which must have been an aborted mission, which meant, maybe, that all those passengers on board had sacrificed themselves, knowing what they were doing, accepting their fate but refusing to give up.

Our first message of condolence came within the hour, and all week others have followed. People have come as individuals and in groups to offer sympathy and express shared horror. Ordinary villagers, neighbors, fellow workers, the authorities one after another. All ask me to tell my countrymen how saddened they are by what happened.

And yet. And yet. Not here, but I know in places, and not so far away, people are dancing. In the streets, some of them; others just in their hearts. The giant has been struck between the eyes, aha! A senator from one of our neighboring Sharia-law states in Nigeria was on the radio today saying that "of course" he doesn't condone such violence but no, America does not have the right to strike back; it should look inward and see how it must change to prevent these things from happening again.

Being far away and listening to international broadcasts we only hear the broad outlines of events. You, over these coming days and weeks and months, must be seeing and hearing and reading about the individuals—the lives lost, children orphaned, families shattered. For this reason only, I think I am glad to be far away and spared that which must be almost unbearable. I cannot imagine how all those thousands of people who have been touched, bludgeoned, by this tragedy are going to pick themselves up, brush themselves off and get on with life.

And finally, more frightening even than what went before is the thought of what could come next. What does Bush mean when he talks about our "resolve to retaliate"? Are we as smart as we think we are? Are we thinking that if we rattle enough swords the bad guys will be served up sweetly on a silver platter? Or are we thinking of mowing down a few more thousand innocent people to get to the cowards hiding behind them? And then what? How many images of dead peasant babies is the world going to tolerate before turning its wrath back on the giant?

No, one more finally. If now we are really going to try to stamp out global terrorism, does this mean that up to now we have not been trying? Have we some magic trick up our sleeve that we have been holding back, some trick that will do the job, that we will perform, finally, now? I know of a country where peoples' mail is routinely opened and telephones are routinely tapped and bandits are hunted down in their homes and shot at 3 o'clock in the morning. In order to keep the peace. A country that has suffered diplomatic contempt, because that is not democracy or freedom or even right. Are we now going to inch our way in that direction?

Wednesday, 19 Sept. A week has passed and that prickly feeling of rawness is no less acute. We try to get the news on BBC or VOA [radio]—reception is uniformly awful—two or three times a day, always at once hopeful and fearful.

There have been some deadly Christian-Muslim confrontations in Nigeria over the past few months, but we have yet to see that sort of idiocy here in Cameroon.

Tuesday, 2 October 2001

Most of September after the 11th was a write-off as, miserably, I could not get the disaster off my mind. It just sat there, like a gargoyle on my shoulder or in my head, looking down, scowling, threatening to pounce, no matter what little or big thing I was doing. All those answerless questions. Matawa came up last weekend, our first contact with Yaoundé since that day, with a few of his cronies, and to our astonishment rather than expressing the slightest concern or even asking if we had lost anyone in the attack, they immediately started taunting us, asking "What are you guys up to over there?" and informing us that "The whole world is laughing at you, you know" and then recounting to one another "humorous" and believe-it-or-not stories of pictures they had seen of people [in New York] trying to flee for their lives through the rubble. Matawa further informed us that "You did it to yourselves" and that Bush himself was behind the attack on the Pentagon, since the Pentagon is "the information center" of the country and "everyone knows" that Bush rigged the election and had to destroy the evidence. All of this was recounted nonstop with the utmost authority, no questions asked, no comment invited, no rebuttal expected. I do not know how representative his feelings are of the feelings of other semi-worldly African Muslims or city folk, but his outpouring reminded me again of how close to the surface is the resentment of America, even among our friends.

Sunday, 7th Oct. AA arrived yesterday afternoon and came over in the evening. He spent a good hour with us, listening and talking calmly about what had happened—[happened] not just to America but to us all, he kept saying. He was concerned that we might be afraid, being here, and for the future and [about] whether our leaders would have the wisdom to do what is right. It was a simple chat, no questions answered, just shared, but it did us both a great deal of good.

Just before and after the start of the new millennium, all of Nigeria's northern states adopted some form of Sharia law, or law based on Quranic teaching. At the hospital we began seeing more female patients garbed in full-length, monochromatic light blue or black veils whose narrow openings exposed only the face, sometimes only the eyes. Crudely drafted and reproduced tracts predicting the downfall of contemporary society and the emergence of an Islamist state were intercepted by Cameroon government authorities, and their distributors were called in for questioning. Nigerian men began carrying plasticized picture ID cards that featured a black flag with white Arabic lettering and declaimed their allegiance to an Islamic fraternity.

Sunday, 04 November 2001

The Sept. 11th attacks remain almost constantly on my mind, no matter what else is happening. So many conflicting thoughts. It seems to me there should be a screeching chorus of prominent Muslims crying out in every language, on every possible podium, that that kind of violence is not what their religion is about. It is not the "west" that should be rallying against the Taliban and their cronies, it is Muslims all over the world whose faith they have stolen and stomped on and smeared with—well, whatever. Why are they so silent? That is what frightens me most of all.

Faith was a force whose strength was impossible to overestimate. We saw this in big ways as in small. At dawn one Tuesday in late April, a twenty-year-old herder knocked at my door. In spite of a tourniquet of cotton cloth belting his right thigh, he stood in a pool of his own blood. An older man I took to be his father was beside him, holding him by an elbow.

I asked the young man to lie down in the sand, and this he did readily before explaining his story to me. The day before, he had gone to a marabout and asked to be given a medicine or charm that would protect him from harm should someone attack him with a knife, an arrow, or a spear. In exchange for a plump chicken, the marabout mixed his potion and the young man drank it. That evening the youth took his dagger and plunged it into his right thigh, confident in his protection and curious to see how the blade would either bend or bounce off. To his astonishment and agony, it did neither.

After ascertaining that the wound, two inches long and several inches deep, had severed no major vessels, I fixed a better bandage on the injured thigh and sent the pair up to the hospital for suturing. Faith in this instance may have done little for the believer, but it was impressive nonetheless.

Every Jutting Rib, Every Mother's Tear

I LOOKED FORWARD longingly to those summers every other year that would give me a break from the relentless tension, pressing demand, and exhausting night calls that defined my life in Kolofata. Once on home turf and surrounded by people I loved, I basked in the contentedness of golden days that passed much too quickly, and leaving them again was never easy. My parents, though in generally good health, were aging, and they and I knew that anything could happen to any of us. That final hug and kiss good-bye always had the sting of understanding that they might be our last ever. Yet I never doubted that I would go back to Cameroon.

By the fall of 2002, the hospital had grown to include six major pavilions. We had electricity, a back-up generator, running water, X-ray and ultrasound, and a satellite phone that allowed us to connect, rudimentarily at least, with the outside world. Beyond the hospital we were taking advantage of a multitude of channels to support education and community development in and around Kolofata. Things were moving forward.

Thursday, 10 October 2002

As much as I miss you, and I do very much, and as much as I miss all that food and comfort and the mindless ease of things that are so difficult or tedious here—I am happy to be back. Every jutting rib, every swollen belly, every feverish cheek, every mother's tear reminds me how happy I am to be back. Sometimes, often, the whole world and all its nonsense seem to distill down to the moment to moment struggle of a sick child fighting for his life.

Sunday, 1st Dec. 2002

Killings took place in Kaduna [Nigeria] this past week in reaction to (as I understand it) a female Christian journalist's having suggested that Mohammed would have been happy to marry one (several?) of the contestants in the Miss World competition which was supposed to have taken place in Abuja, the capital. In response to this perceived insult, fundamentalists went on the rampage, slaughtering hundreds. Here is where the culture gap is abysmal and terrifying: My reaction on hearing this news was to wonder in horror and dismay how a peaceful people—during the most disciplined and peaceful month of their year— could respond in such a violent and, to my mind, wildly inappropriate way to this slight, if that's what it was. However, the episode has come up twice, briefly, in discussions with others here—both men, both Muslims, both moderately educated. Their one and only remark was—She shouldn't have written what she wrote. Not a hint of condemnation for the killers. I know there will never be peace in the world, but you just wish sometimes that there could be a little less stupidity.

Saturday, 29 March 2003

I should be 1) doing laundry, 2) cleaning the bathroom, 3) cleaning period or 4) preparing meetings, and so I think I will start a letter. That will give me time to reflect on which of the above I should attack first. We have had a busy and tiring week, bookended by middle-of-the-night deliveries of twins. The first, Monday night, were premature stillborn girls. My worry in that case was not the babies but the mother who had complications, including premature detachment of the placenta, but our luck held and we got through the ordeal unscathed.

Last night's started in the morning when I was called because a woman in labor had just come in and the baby's umbilical cord had slipped out before the baby. The baby was breech, the first of twins. There was a feeble pulse in the cord, but as we encouraged the mother to push (the cervix was fully dilated) the pulse disappeared and failed to come back after the contraction ceased. I had no choice but to try to force the delivery, and in so doing I broke the baby's left arm—oh, what an awful sound and awful feeling, that krack under your fingers. We got her out and she was not breathing but she was not dead and the resuscitation was not difficult. We splinted her arm and she seemed to take it all in stride and since then has appeared to be unfazed by it. Her little sister, having telepathically understood, perhaps, what dangers awaited her, was in no hurry to come down. She was also breech, in a second amniotic sac.

It happened that Kolofata was receiving a [government] minister and my presence was required all afternoon and evening at an official ceremony and reception. He was the minister of education but had previously been minister of health and had been in Kolofata in 1995 to inaugurate one of our buildings. After the ceremonious garbage, I went back up to check on the woman in labor, and she was as I had left her—stable, waters unbroken, baby hanging back. Came home, went to bed, was called again at 10, just as I had closed my book (about the 1949 pennant race between the Red Sox and the Yankees, and it is fun, especially at this particular time when the world is such a mess: helps to remind me of what is really important in life). Not, it turned out, for the lady in labor but for another who had just come in hemorrhaging from a miscarriage.

This woman was pouring out blood as if there were a spigot up there with a cross-threaded tap that wouldn't turn off. Terrifying thoughts pound in my head—and they are terrifying and they do pound; it is like being in the middle of a raging thunderstorm all alone in the middle of nowhere, and sometimes I have to look up to realize, with astonishment always, that the room is so still and quiet you can hear a graceful lizard brush against the floor—and the thoughts are along these lines: Am I watching this woman live the last five minutes of her life? If I don't do something or do do something else, will her children never see their mother again? And all the while I am giving orders to the nurse—position the patient, give the injection, start the IV—and going through the motions— clamp down on the uterus, set the speculum, scoop out the debris—with a methodical deliberateness I do not feel. (What I feel is like shouting at the #@ lX! blood to turn off.)

She did fine, but it was not easy. I would no sooner think that I had gotten it all than she would start bleeding again and I'd have to go back in and I'd find some tiny scrap of ratty placenta that had clung on and been left behind. So when I'd finished with her I went to check on our lady in labor.

All was as we had left it except the first twin was getting hungry and the mother was getting tired and discouraged. The second twin had come down, so I went ahead and broke the waters and a half hour later delivered the baby— breech, but this one, though bigger, was easy. No broken bones. When I looked up after clamping the cord, the grandmother and aunt, who had been the woman's faithful helpers and moral supporters, had tears streaming down their faces. I got the baby squared away and then looking up over her still bulging belly asked the mother if she had any more left in there. No, she said, that would be enough for now.

The children's ward is close enough to being finished that I think we are going to move in this coming week.

Wednesday, 23 April 2003

[A] 39 year old man [with leprosy] felt an itch on his left foot, the sole. He put it near the fire and that seemed to calm the itch so nicely that he moved it a little

closer. In fact quite close. Then he smelled roasting meat. One of the things lep-
rosy does is destroy peripheral nerves, so patients lose feeling in their hands and
feet. This young man came to us with a four inch hole burned into the bottom of
his foot. The big toe was burned right off.

Thursday, 29 May 2003

[A] storm rolled in and unleashed our first real rain of the season. Our roof
[at home] leaked like a sieve. We were tripping over ourselves trying to get bowls
under the streams of water falling from a dozen different points in the ceiling. We
would no sooner get one covered than the thunk-thunk-thunk-swoosh of another
leak somewhere else would begin. The lights had gone off, of course, and with the
storm it was dark outside and darker inside. This house is chock-a-block full of
papers—files, letters, magazines, journals, photos, books—and there is nothing
like a leaky roof to make us realize how fragile is the stuff of our existence.

Some Day My Very Soul Will Leave My Body

THE OLD INTRIGUED me. They were calm. Their blurry eyes had seen so much. By
and large they were without guile and had nothing left to prove, whether to themselves or to others. Their vaunted wisdom came from this, perhaps, and also from
the fact that they were still upright after so many decades of being buffeted about.

An elderly gentleman came to us one afternoon suffering much pain from a
bladder that would not empty. We inserted a Foley catheter, a tube whose tip
encloses a deflated balloon that we fill with water once the catheter is inside the
bladder. About chestnut size when inflated, this balloon ensures that the catheter
will not slip out until it is purposely deflated again.

Over the next couple of days, our patient decided he no longer liked being connected to this tube and asked me to take it out. I did not refuse, but I told him
I did not think it was a good idea to remove it quite yet, and I explained to him
why we wanted to leave it in for a few more days. He nodded to convey that he
had heard me, but I noted that he professed neither agreement nor dissent, and
the next morning on rounds we found the catheter, covered with blood, lying on
the mat beside him.

"It fell out," he said.

The balloon was still inflated to capacity, so it could not have fallen out, especially given the size of his bloated prostate. Someone had had to yank it out, and
I guessed that someone was him.

"How could it have fallen out?" I asked, making no attempt to hide my disbelief.

"Ha!" he answered. "Some day my very soul will leave my body. Why not a rubber tube today?" He was not displeased with himself.

I entertained a hope that he might have unwittingly enlarged the urethral passage, but he went back into retention within hours, and in the afternoon when I offered to replace the catheter until we could send him for surgery, he accepted gladly.

Later that day a Fulani woman came into my consulting room. She had cotton-white hair and an exotically scarred face with more folds and furrows than a walnut shell. Like many old women around Kolofata, she wore a black net cap under a black velvet bonnet. Her dress was black crepe with white geometric designs at the bodice and sleeves, and covering it from the waist down was a purple wrapper shot with shiny silver threads. A black velvet shawl with long fringe draped her shoulders, and molded plastic vividly purple shoes encased her feet. A silver loop hung from each earlobe, whose holes were stretched to slits an inch long. Globular silver rings had somehow slipped over the arthritic joints of her fingers. A dozen bangle bracelets clanged on both arms. On the left they fought for pride of place with a black plastic watch whose face proclaimed "Sporty Casual" in white curlicue letters. However intriguingly glamorous, I guessed she was a great-grandmother many times over.

I jotted down her name and the name of her village and then, "How old are you?" I asked.

She smiled and paused to think. The measurement of age was an odd Western preoccupation, so the question was probably one she had never been asked. She looked at me with some bewilderment at first, and then, "Twenty-five," she replied with no hint that she meant anything else.

I nodded, glanced sideways at her to make sure she was not just teasing me, and wrote *60*.

Tuesday, 17 June 2003

   I have been in my first tornado.

   Saturday evening around 6:30 we had finished eating and could tell there was a storm coming, so I let Myra handle the dishes while I set up my satellite phone and computer out front in an effort to get my e-mailing in before the rain. The sky in the east was dark, but there wasn't much wind yet, and no drops. But I'd just gotten the phone set up and turned on when a terrific roar started moving in from that darkened east. Sometimes a rainstorm starts like that—but in that case you can hear the drops of rainfall moving curtainlike toward you, and the sound is loud, but nothing like this. I hurriedly scooped up my equipment—not having yet made a connection—and scuttled inside and at the same time Myra was scuttling in through the back door. The storm hit, swirling black winds, thunder, lightning, pelting rain. The worst—we did not yet know how bad—was over in a matter of minutes at most. The rain continued more gently for another 20 or 30 minutes. Then we went out to take a look. Oh la la. Mature trees pulled up by their roots, others topped or missing thick branches, roofs torn off, walls toppled, electric poles down and wires trailing across almost every street. A galvanized steel pipe attached to our own house—it once held an antenna on top—was bent like a paper matchstick. People recounted having been levitated. We were lucky. No deaths, and apart from a few patients who came with cuts, scrapes and bruises, no serious injuries. Massive branches had been torn off the trees I park my Land Rover under, and they lay on the ground nestling against it on three sides, but it did not have a scrape or a dent anywhere. Our house was fine, and the hospital as well, in spite of all the half-trees lying about. One of our nurses lost his house, but he was renting, so apart from the inconvenience of rescuing wet papers and clothes and having to find new lodging it's not too bad. His wife and child were out of town visiting her mother at the time—another blessing, because the roof fell in on him. He is a big strong guy and suffered scrapes and bruises; his wife and baby might not have been so lucky. All Saturday night and Sunday and yesterday and today we hear pounding pounding pounding: people with axes chopping fallen branches into hangar poles and firewood, and others replacing doors and windows and roofs. Everyone I have talked to says they have never seen anything like it, so I figure chances are good it will never happen to us again, which is a comforting thought. The electricity is out, of course.

Tuesday, 9 Sept. 2003

One of my patients today was an 8 month old malnourished baby, all ribs, pointy joints, swollen feet and skin sores. She was in the arms of her mother, a woman of about 16, and she was accompanied by a garrulous grey-haired man who assured me he was not the father of the child but rather of the mother. Where, I asked, is the child's father?

"Ha"—the old man gave a gesture of dismissal—"he ran away. He got her pregnant and then he ran away. Lagos. She delivered in my own house. Now look what I am left with. Nothing but suffering. How could she go and marry a Nigerian?"

Well, I said, you are her father, why did you give her to a Nigerian?

"Did I give her?" he asked. "She went. She wanted that Nigerian boy. Got her pregnant and then ran away."

Coming back to the problem at hand, I asked the mother, Is she sucking? She said no. Why? I asked. She looked at me coyly. Paused. Said, "I'm pregnant." Oh, I said, how many months? "Four, five." I looked at the father.

"Yes," he despaired. "You see what a Nigerian will do?"

If the Nigerian ran away to Lagos, how is it she is pregnant again?

"Maybe he came back—do I know what happens when I am not at home? You see how I suffer so much?"

How many children do you have?

He didn't even have to think. "Thirty-five. Four wives. I suffer. I suffer."

Who forced you to marry four wives? I asked.

He stared back as if it were the first time he had considered the question. "Well," he shrugged, "yes," and said no more.

The child if she lives will be with us for some time.

Saturday, 27 September 2003

This week I got a patient, seven months old, [whose] neck was festooned with tiny animal paws and hoofs strung on a leather thong. There must have been a dozen or fifteen species hanging there—various bush rats and rabbits and I don't know porcupines and maybe goat or sheep fetuses. Hoofs and claws, fur and bones, cloven and not. Often children have two or three such animal parts—paws, claws, birds' heads and the like—dangling round their necks, but this was the first time I saw a child with a whole menagerie. The father a hunter perhaps.

Just Weeds

Sunday, 7th Dec. 2003

[One morning this week] a woman in her late 30s came in bleeding to death after having partially expelled a molar pregnancy. I had to leave rounds to tend to her, [empty] her uterus, find a donor and get fresh blood going into her.

Meanwhile an Italian nun of 55 or 60 came in near to fainting with a 105 degree temperature and a case of malaria that she had been trying—unsuccessfully, clearly—to treat at various hospitals elsewhere. She informed me she was going to faint. She is a stoutish woman, and no sooner had I got her on the table than she clutched her chest and informed me that now she was going to die. She was grunting ominously and muttering incoherently something about her mother, and she probably did not hear me but I informed her back that there was no way an Italian nun was going to die in my hospital.

Then the sous-préfet was announced at my back door. Usually he would call me up to see him in his office or he would send a minion down with whatever problem or file or paper he wanted to present. The fact that he had come himself meant that he considered his business high priority, so I quickly went to the door to tell him that I had an emergency on my hands and I would be a few minutes, but before I could close the door on him he just wanted to present the problem, which consisted of a request that I falsify a report in order to get some funds released from the Treasury. (I can't do that, I said. Yes you can, he replied: This is Africa. No, I said, I really really cannot do that.) And by the way he wanted these papers photocopied please. The hospital is the only place in town that has a photocopier. All government services are provided with money for that sort of thing, but the hospital, in its un-African naïveté, is the only one that uses it for that. I apologized, told him he would have to leave them, I had an emergency I was worried about, and good-bye for now, I would get back to him.

We got the nun carried by stretcher to a room and an IV and medicines [going] into her. As we were doing that a man rushed in with a transfer note from one of our health centers. He had brought a woman 8 months pregnant suffering agitation or convulsions for the past 3 days. She was sprawled uneasily under a tree outside my consulting room. As soon as the nun was squared away I brought her in and tried to figure out if this new woman was genuinely sick or faking it—it turned out to be mostly the latter, but it is time consuming to settle on that conclusion and meanwhile there were the distraught relatives who were miffed and panicked by the alternating states of catatonia and dramatic "seizures" they were witnessing in their loved one.

At the same time a contractor was there to install our big generator—the one that was supposed to have been installed a year ago, but that contractor had a motorcycle accident, broke his leg in several places, had no luck with the aftermath and remains largely out of commission. With unfathomable stupidity, we (I) had already paid him for the installation (he was working on it when he had his accident) and I had hoped he would do the right thing and see to it that the job got done, but after a year of hoping I gave up. Anyway, the new contractor was turning the lights on and off and he was in and out asking for keys and parts and so on, and this was not on the whole helpful at that time. The upshot of that story is that a piece of the new generator is defective and has to be replaced—the coil rewound—and as I write we remain uninstalled.

While I was with the pregnant lady, a nurse from another of our health centers came by with a couple of problems, one of which was that he wanted to borrow an AIDS video, since it was national AIDS week and [there] was going to be a movie night and roundtable at the health center. Unfortunately the nurse in charge of our book and video library was on holiday that day so I—eventually Myra—had to scramble around to find where this particular video was kept etc.

Little things, but everything takes time, and meanwhile there is a room full of patients wondering what is taking me so long to get to them, and I am feeling bad because they are waiting so patiently and because I wonder how I am going to wade through that whole crowd and get to the end of the day.

That was how the week went, more or less. Mostly more. The nun did fine.

Sunday, 14 December 2003

[A] mobile phone relay has been installed in Mora, and it is said that there are places in Kolofata where reception is possible. Our compound is not one of these places, but the hospital up on the hill is. So we are busy investigating possibilities, and it might just be that soon we will enter into some kind of credible communication network with the rest of the country—and beyond.

Saturday, 03 January 2004

So we have a cell phone, "temporarily." AA brought it up for us, already set up and accessorized with spare calling cards, gave it to us "temporarily" which means (as with tennis rackets and VCR and satellite dish and house) for as long as we care to use it here.

30 year old Nigerian man walks into the consulting room.

Pt: Madame. I want test my power here (pointing to scale).
Dr: Okay. (Pt. gets on scale.) 69 kg.
Pt: Is good?
Dr: Very good.
Pt (smiling): Yah, that's good all right.

Too often during the cold harmattan months, when people were so desperate to get warm that they huddled around wood or reed fires, inching ever forward to better absorb the heat, hungry flames would lick at a corner of their cloth and in a flash go on to consume the rest of it and them. Children and the elderly were particularly vulnerable.

In January an old woman, Aissa, came to us with third-degree burns over much of the front part of her body. Her entire hut and everything in it, and the huts on either side of hers, had burned down. Recovery from serious burns was a long and painful ordeal that involved daily unwrapping of dressings, disinfection, debriding, and agonizing physiotherapy aimed at keeping joints as supple as possible.

On rounds one morning, Aissa, desiccated as a mummy, was lying so still that we approached her thinking she was dead. Gingerly I folded back her blanket and was relieved to see her chest moving. When I shook her and called her name, her gummy trachomatous half-blind eyes flickered. The nurse going off night duty informed me that the family had come to him in the night to tell him that Aissa had died. When he went to her room to investigate, the nurse found her much as we were finding her now. He said he had succeeded in rousing her, and she had told him she was hungry. He had given her a light porridge, and by the time she had finished drinking it she was sitting up and looking almost perky. This morning as we roused her she again said that she was hungry. I asked the two daughters and husband who were staying with her what they had to eat.

"Nothing," they replied.

"Nothing?" I asked. "What does that mean? What did you eat yesterday?"

They looked at me sheepishly but did not reply. I pushed.

"Food," they said at last.

"What kind of food?" I asked.

One of the daughters went to a corner of the room and picked up a canvas sack that had a few cupfuls of millet flour in the bottom of it.

"This," they said. "It's all we saved from the fire."

"Well," I said, "but what kind of sauce. What did you put in the sauce?"

They would not answer. I turned to Aissa. "Aissa, what kind of sauce did you have yesterday?"

She looked at her daughters, not wanting to reply. I insisted, confused. "What kind of sauce?" I asked again.

"Weeds," she said. "Just weeds." No one contradicted her.

"OK," I said. "But oil too? Dried fish? Beans?"

"Just weeds," she said again, pointing to the field.

We rectified that problem immediately. But I cringed to realize she would have died, and I would never have known that her death was not from her wounds but from starvation.

People Say It Is Blood Being Poured Over the Moon

Thursday, 26 February 2004

This morning I rounded for the first time on a 60 year old Nigerian man who walks, barely, with a beautifully carved cane and who weighs 75 pounds. He was admitted yesterday by the nurse for a cough of three years' duration. As I was examining him, one of the nurses behind me remarked, "He brought his burial cloth." I looked over to the end of his bed and saw a neat bundle of white cloth bound with a white cloth cord beside his pillow, as if he wanted to be sure it was well within reach. He was all ribs and knobby knees and because the fat had gone from his face, his ears stuck out from the sides of his head and he looked like a mouse in a world without cheese. We tested him for TB and he was positive. By the end of the day he was started on treatment and I told him his chances of being well again were good. He should hold on to the cloth, for one day he would surely need it, but not yet I did not think.

We finally said good-bye to a patient, a man of about 35, who had come to us from Lagos to be treated. Lagos is the former capital of Nigeria, a gigantic city, one of the biggest in the world, filled [with] and surrounded by teaching hospitals, and it is located approximately six zillion miles from here. This man had been sick for a long time with heart and renal failure. He could hardly breathe, and he could not walk, and he was so edematous it looked like he'd do better to roll rather than walk from one place to another anyway. I cannot imagine how news of Kolofata reached him in Lagos, but it did, and clearly whoever brought it to him recounted tales of miracles, for he and his wife convinced her brother, who has a car, to make the four-day journey up-country and across the border to seek out this fabled hospital. The brother dropped them off and the next day turned around and went back to Lagos. I believe he was sure it was the last he would see of his brother-in-law and he was probably congratulating himself for having escaped funeral duties and expenses. Had I known he was from Lagos, I would not have let the wife's brother leave, for I, too, thought our patient would most likely die and having a total stranger with no family die in hospital is a hassle. But amazingly, he did not die, he did well, quite well in fact, and after ten days I told them they would be going home. That was when I learned that home was Lagos and that they would have to wait for the brother to come back to get them—not for another few days, the wife thought. A few days then turned into a few more days and then a few weeks and eventually they were turning into permanent residents. We were frustrated because we needed the bed; they were frustrated because they wanted to go home—and maybe because they started to wonder if the family had planned all along to dump them. Only once in every 7 or 8 days could the wife get a telephone call to go through. Eventually she found some brave soul who lent her the money for them to get back to Lagos by public transportation, and off they finally went. The patient was fine, but he'll need follow-up. I hope he finds someone a little closer to home.

We did not see many cases of rape. I doubted this was because rape was rare but rather because in general it was not considered to be much of a problem, medical or otherwise. If a girl was raped and the rapist was found out, he was encouraged or forced to marry the girl or else settle with the girl's father on a hefty sum for having, as they put it, destroyed her.

In one of our cases, the accused rapist was a repeat offender, and the village had finally tired of his hijinks. The girl was eight years old, and a tiny eight at that, and the rapist tore her vagina badly enough that she trailed a pool of blood as she waddled home. An orphan, she was being raised by an uncle and grandmother who preferred to keep her at home to do chores rather than send her to school. The accused was a neighbor, a young man. The girl claimed that she was fetching firewood in a field when he came up on his bicycle, accosted her, tackled her, and stuffed her headscarf in her mouth. When he had finished with her, he told her he would kill her if she breathed a word of it. He rode back to the village and went straight to the girl's uncle to explain that he had had a bicycle accident and toppled his niece, who did not seem to be badly hurt, though she was bleeding a little and he was awfully sorry.

Possibly the girl had intended to keep her attacker's secret, but when the uncle saw her straggle home, he realized what had happened and brought her to see me. I examined her tattered tissues, ran the requisite tests, and wrote my report. The police issued a warrant for the man's arrest, and the village chief brought him in the next day.

When I went to see the police chief so that I could get an HIV test on the prisoner, I was surprised to find the chief amused that the family was pressing charges.

"If he refuses to marry the girl," the officer explained, "then maybe I could understand. But why doesn't he just agree to marry her and the problem is over?"

I pointed out that the girl was eight years old.

He shrugged. "Still," he said.

I asked him if rape was not a crime in Cameroon.

He assured me that it was. "But we never see it. The families always manage to work things out."

This family had no interest in working anything out. The rapist went to prison and stayed there. For three months.

Sunday, May 9, 2004

On May 4th 2004 at 7:48 PM local time we started watching a full eclipse of the moon. The sky was perfectly clear and the gradual and inexorable veiling of the moon was one of the spookiest things I have ever seen. The people say it is blood being poured over the moon and it is God showing his power and warning that he is going to lash out. As soon as the veil started to draw closed, old women all over town started beating buckets and pots and basins with sticks and begging for mercy and forgiveness, and children ganged together and started parading through town chanting verses from the Quran, and the men gathered in the mosque and furiously fingered their prayer beads, and all of this went on until the early hours of the morning when the moon at last gave us back his light. I sat in our front courtyard and watched for the hour or so it took for the brilliant full moon to be transformed to a barely smoldering orange disk, and then I went to bed, trusting the old women to bang hard and loud and long enough to protect us all.

Nearly three years later, at one o'clock in the morning, someone would discover that the moon was again "not working right," and the town would be awakened by marabouts calling for women to pound pots and men to pray. I remember thinking, even in the middle-of-the-night haze of my brain, how perfect that was, that when stakes were high, men were expected to count beads and women to move the moon.

God Decided Her Time Had Come to Die

Saturday, 13 November 2004

Happy Ramadan! We went over to see Mme. Ali [who has come from Yaoundé] this morning and she had been up much of the night organizing the kitchen staff (and I gather all night saying things like "What do you mean, we have no knives?" and "What do you mean, the firewood is all gone?" and "Why is that bull still not slaughtered?"). She has to put together a massive meal for hundreds, and I do not envy her the job. This morning she was obsessed with potatoes—I don't know, but I'm guessing fifty or sixty pounds—that were still not peeled. Every time Moussa or one of the kitchen staff came into the house hoisting a platter or pot, she put the question to them: Are the potatoes peeled yet? The answer was uniformly vague. At first the potatoes could not be found. Then they were checking into it. Then someone thought someone or other was getting ready to attack them. Eventually we did hear from one of the girls that she did think, or she was pretty sure, the potatoes were getting peeled. Mme. Ali finally excused herself and said it was time she go out and see how things were going back there!

Everyone is in new clothes, clean and shiny, and there is a holiday shimmer in the air. Someone just brought over a huge platter laden with rice and meat sauce and a roasted chicken and deep-fried cookies, plus we will probably be going over to feast with AA, so we are being looked after and included in the happy festivities. I can't wait to see how the potatoes turned out.

Later. Just fine, as it happens. We had a lovely meal, ate till our bellies ached, and then forced down a glass of champagne. Well, Myra forced down three—unless there were one or two in between that I didn't see—and declared it a perfectly satisfying meal.

Sunday, 10 April 2005.

We are thinking that [a] guy whose hand we saved last weekend is probably a member of a gang of cattle rustlers or thieves, and we are fixing him up to go rob another day. Unless he turns out to be like Jean Valjean. He smokes Benson & Hedges—I have twice confiscated the gold packs and lighter—and slinks off to heaven knows where for hours at a time, and he has a disarming smile and careful gaze, like that of a hunter on tenterhooks looking and listening for [the] telltale snap of a twig. He wears a copper ring on the second toe of his right foot, and we are all sure that means something. And the thin, turbaned fellows who come to see him are as mysterious and expert at avoiding telling you where they are from. It is Nigeria one day, Niger the next, a finger pointing vaguely to the south the next. They wear indigo robes with long knives under them strapped at their waists and plastic shoes on their feet. One of them, coming up to me yesterday to ask me a question, addressed me—"Hey, Fulani Woman!" I said, "Hey, Fulani Man, what?"

So vital was breastmilk to the survival of an infant in poor African communities that the death of a mother within the first year of her newborn's life was almost inevitably a death sentence for the child as well. Tinned infant formula was outrageously expensive, no other nutritionally adequate substitute was locally available, safe drinking water was rare, and fathers lacked the time and expertise to raise a baby. For these reasons, even if the father was alive, it was common to call motherless infants "orphans." We developed a program whereby we provided orphans with tinned formula and health care if extended family members were able to bring the child every couple of weeks to the hospital while otherwise caring for him or her at home.

Thursday, 8 September 2005

We seem to be having an epidemic of orphans these days, which is to say a lot of young mothers [must be] dying soon after childbirth. This may be the downside of the rainy season and all those impassable roads. Or it may be because people are poor this time of year (the harvest is not in for another month or two) [and] do not want to spend money on hospital care. The story is always more or less the same. The mother delivered at home, she bled heavily, she died the next day. Or she delivered at home, she got fever, and the next week she died. Sometimes it's all I can do to keep myself from punching the husband who recounts such a tale to me. Why did you not bring her to hospital when you saw there was a problem? I ask over and over, and the answer only infuriates me further. "I wasn't at home," he says, "so she had no money to go to hospital." That is by far the most common answer. I count to ten. "Your wife is at term with your child. You know she is at term with your child. You take off. Fine. How can you not leave some money with her or with a brother or a neighbor in case something goes wrong?" He shrugs (which means exactly this: God decided her time had come to die, so she died. There's nothing I could have done to save my wife. I can't go against God) and mutters something about next time . . . and I'm thinking, Next time! That's just great! And really the urge to do something violent to this [fellow] is just this side of overwhelming. Today we got day-old twins, a boy and a girl. A village only about 7 km from here. The mother delivered at home, she bled, the father had vanished several days earlier, leaving no money. The dead mother's sister brought the babies to us this morning, hoping we might be able to help with milk.

They Close the Nose and Mouth, Lest the Last Breath Escape

Sunday, 11 December 2005

[I sent our two American] medical students out Friday with two of the polio vaccination teams [to] give them the chance to participate in this history-making disease eradication process. I assigned them to Kolofata. They were each the 3rd man on a 2-man team, so their work was not arduous and it was the nurses who carried the heavy thermoses and other gear [door-to-door]. Nevertheless, the day exhausted them and I wish you could have seen them as they stumbled home eleven hours later, barely able to walk, covered in dust, [one] saying, "Kolofata is just about the biggest city I have ever seen in my whole life." They threw themselves into chairs, slumped and crumpled, and I wondered if they would find the strength to rise again. A few moments later their [Cameroonian] teammates strolled in, bright-eyed and beaming, their white coats still glowing as if they had just come from the wash. They smiled wryly when they saw their defeated comrades.

January 21, 2006

A case of rabies earlier in the week. A young, fit man of about 30, bitten by a dog two months ago. If some day I have to die—and the evidence is fairly convincing that I do—I do not want to die of rabies. Air hunger and water phobia. Fierce random spasms make you gasp and choke uncontrollably. You are hungry and thirsty but cannot eat or drink. You are tired—exhausted—and cannot sleep, cannot rest. Every neuron is on full alert. You see everything, feel everything, know everything. As if you had drunk gallons of strong black coffee. You cannot sleep, not for one minute, and this goes on for four, five, six days until at last you expire from exhaustion. We had him on 8 times the maximum dose of sedatives that I would normally put an adult on, and it did not touch him. I would have kept going up and up, but the family opted to carry him home to die in his village. I hope they have some leaves and roots there that will do a better job than our pharmaceuticals.

Monday, 2 May 2006

Last Saturday evening the American ambassador and his 2nd consul came up and stayed until Monday morning. His name is Neils Marquardt, a towering blond Dane. I'm sure his ancestors were Vikings. My age. Speaks excellent French. Smiles a lot. Seems interested in everything. Wore a flowing Muslim outfit the first day, complete with little embroidered cap, and a sports shirt and baseball hat the second day—the perfect diplomat! We had a nice dinner Saturday night and a full day Sunday, a blazing hot sunny day. After breakfast we went to meet AA's father—at 95 and the oldest man in town, he is a tourist attraction after all—then did tours of the Women's Center and the hospital. After that we went out to a few villages where AA has his mango orchards and a number of experimental farms—one a date palm grove, another a vineyard, another the start of what he hopes will be a fish farm. He (AA) is full of ideas and thinks that nothing is impossible, and he was in fine form showing all this off and expounding at length with the ambassador, who could not have been a more enthusiastic listener. It was around 2 PM when we got back to Kolofata and had another lavish meal. The ambassador and I went out to play tennis. He beat me in a tiebreaker the first set and was up 3-2 when we had to stop because it was getting too dark for aging eyes. It was great fun.

Tuesday, 14 November 2006

A woman in her 8th pregnancy came in at 8 months after having been bleeding at home for several days. The day before she had bled a lot and noticed that the baby had stopped moving. By the time she got to us, she was weak from blood loss and unable to stand or even sit without fainting. I was horrified to [find] her sitting on the floor in a corner of the [delivery] room, propped up by five other women. [One held] a green cloth over our patient's nose and mouth, effectively smothering her. The dead fetus, still sealed in his intact amniotic pouch, the placenta riding along that like a backpack, lay on the floor beside her in a pond of blood and blood clots. My first thought was: This is how they kill them; this is how they die. All those mothers of all those orphans we keep getting, when the hard-to-believe story is so often that "She delivered and then she just died."

I shouted at the women to lay her down, while doing so myself against their resistance, and I grabbed the green smothering cloth from her face. One woman grabbed it back and tried to cover the nose and mouth again, pleading, The air, the air! I snatched it and threw it down with a fury and chased the whole lot of them out of the room. Got the woman down with her feet up and cleaned the clots out of her uterus while clamping down on it with one hand. [I] bloodied my phone calling for two nurses and we got fluid racing into her and the woman, who regained consciousness as soon as she was lying down and freed of the green cloth, in spite of the pain she was in, kept saying thank you thank you thank you. She did fine. Four days later she walked out of the hospital.

Tuesday, 12 December 2006

So desperate are we to see some sign of Christmas that when we watch the news on CNN we scan the screen and rejoice when we see, for example, pine branches strewn across the mantle at the White House, or a store decorated in the background of a street shot, or a woman with a holiday brooch.

Friday I was called for a woman in labor with her 9th child. A Nigerian. A ninth baby should slide as easily as a trombone, but this one's head was not flexed properly so every time the mother pushed, the baby's head just jammed up against her pelvic bones and he went nowhere. She was short. Her co-wife was in the room with her, comforting her and encouraging her and seeming at least as distraught as the woman herself. I sized up the situation—woman stable, baby alive, head high, cervix fully dilated, vulva massively edematous from all the manipulation that had been done in the village—and left the room to fetch the vacuum. I learned later that my leaving the room upset them—"The doctor just came; why is she leaving, can nothing be done?"—until the nurse reassured them. We got the cup on the baby's head and pumped up the pressure and pulled—but I got the angle wrong, and that attempt failed. Tried again, and this time it was right. In one little pop that I could feel though not hear, the head came unwedged and out the little guy came. Not so little—10½ pounds, which here puts him into the giant class. He wriggled right away and screamed soon after, unscathed by the trauma, unmoved by the drama. The co-wife came right over to me as I still had the baby suspended by the ankles and she wrapped her arms around me, tears in her eyes.

Sunday, 7 January 2007

Yesterday as I was coming down from the hospital I came upon a traditional healer also coming down. He had his jug of brownish liquid with a dispensing cup attached to it by a cord. We were only about 20 meters outside the hospital gate, on the path that leads nowhere but to [and from] the hospital. I stopped, greeted him, asked him how he was, asked him what he was up to. No, no, he said immediately. I wasn't coming from there. By which I understood that he was most certainly coming from there. I'm not sure whether he had clandestinely made the rounds of our patients or whether he sort of set up shop at the gates to solicit patients coming or going. I nodded and smiled and bid him good day.

Tuesday, 23 January 2007

The call a few nights ago was for a convulsing 3 year old. By the time I got to him he was barely alive. His mother insisted on holding her hand over his face, the way they do, smothering him. As soon as I got into the room I grabbed her wrist and pulled it away. She wriggled it free from my grasp and went back to smothering her son. His eyes rolled back into his head, he was still convulsing, jerking ominously. I grabbed her hand again; she freed it once more and clasped it over the boy's nose and mouth. One last time I pulled it away—I was just about ready to break it off at this point—and wedged it under her so she was sitting on it and I raised my voice and let her know she was not going to win this one. Within a minute of being allowed to breathe, the boy stopped convulsing. His color returned, his body relaxed. Seeing this made a believer of the mother, who was amazed and grateful, and when in the night her son briefly convulsed one last time (it was a case of cerebral malaria) she called the nurse but made no effort to cover his face.

And I really do wonder how many people we lose each year because of this gesture. I bet it is hundreds. They close the nose and mouth to keep life from leaving the body. It makes sense, doesn't it. As long as the nose and mouth are firmly sealed, that last breath cannot escape and therefore the person cannot die. When in spite of their best effort the person dies anyway, they think they reacted too late to seal off the airway or they did not clamp down hard enough. The mother I am sure believed I was killing her child, as surely as I knew she was doing just that.

~⁓

Bodies Lying Contorted on the Sand

Sunday, 4 February 2007

AA came last night. He has been in the news a lot lately. In his position as Minister of Justice he has been shaking things up down there, opening investigations into all sorts of things and going after untouchables. The latest mini saga had to do with prison guards who went on an illegal strike. He fired the lot of them and within a day had new ones recruited and on the job. He is exposing corruption in many sectors that people have known about but done nothing to stop for years. I gather he is making a lot of enemies and hope he is watching his back.

Thursday, 1 March 2007

Last week we had a boy of about 17 with a fractured femur. The bone was broken clean through at mid shaft and the down part was rotated such that the foot looked like it was on the wrong leg. The boy was a would-be goat thief [and] he and a buddy had surreptitiously secreted 13 goats out of various herds and were in the process of trying to snatch three more from another herd when the owner realized what was going on. He came after the buddy first. The owner, bigger than the boy, was unarmed. The thief had a knife, and while they grappled, he thrust it into the back of the goat owner. The man's cries were enough to alert the village, and they took off after the boy, catching him and flogging him thoroughly with branches cut from a thorn tree. The other boy, fleeter of foot and not delayed by a grapple with the owner, took off like a shot and might have escaped had he not tripped off the end of a little bridge and come crashing down with a snapped femur. The villagers soon came upon him, in all their branch-brandishing fury, and ordered him to get up. He tried valiantly and only crumpled back to the ground. They ordered him again. He crumpled again. So it dawned on the good citizens what the problem was and they set to laughing at the fine justice of the thing. The man who had been stabbed in the back was first to arrive in hospital. We patched him up, held on to him for a few days to be sure his lung was okay, then released him. The police brought the boys. The thorn-whipped boy was bloody, swollen and sore, but in no danger. The broken femur boy needed surgery to tack the broken bits back together.

Here is where the story gets sad. He is from a herding tribe who normally are thick as thieves. Nor is it too much to interpret that literally. They are Arab Choas [Choa is the French rendition of Shuwa] and whenever there is one Arab Choa on bed you are sure to find half a dozen or more around taking care of him. They are very devoted to their own and in general mix little with others. But they have a tradition of outlawing. Even young boys wear knives, and they learn at an early age how to wield them. The girls undergo ritual excision (we just got a girl in this week who was bleeding uncontrollably from an amputated clitoris) at about 8 years old—the only tribe left here who do that. Many make their living as cattle, goat and sheep rustlers, and although I've never heard it stated as such, I think teenagers—boys—are expected to enrich the family herd in this way before they can be considered men.

This boy, our fractured femur, was promptly abandoned by everyone. His family, his chief, his village—all stayed away. No one would hand over five francs to even buy him an aspirin. His male relatives (his father is dead; he was raised by an uncle) and chief were summoned by the police to the hospital the night he was brought in and they all made the right sounds about how they were going back to the village to get money and women to stay with the boy and they would be right back, etc. But they left and never came back, despite further summons by the police. The boy with his broken leg languished alone for 3 days. Relatives of other patients around him did what they could, sharing their food and water, helping him when he needed to urinate. It was astonishing to me to see Arab Choas behave this way, and I do not know whether it was because other family members or villagers were involved in the attempted theft and were afraid of being arrested or because they had decided collectively to make an example of a boy who had failed. On the third night he disappeared—presumably they came under cover of darkness and snatched him away. They might take him to a traditional healer, but barring a miracle he will never walk again.

Sometimes during the hot season sleeping was so difficult that I was almost relieved to be called at night. Calls got me out of the stifling house and into the slightly cooler air, and that was refreshing.

One such call on a hot night at the end of March was for a seven-year-old girl brought to us in a deep coma. She had no fever and I saw no sign of trauma. Her breathing was easy and regular, so I thought she might have suffered a stroke but suspected it was more likely that she had been drugged. These suspicions were reinforced when I flashed a light in her eyes and saw her tiny pupils.

The father told me that his daughter had eaten a dinner of millet with gumbo sauce around six thirty that evening and then gone to an uncle's house a block away. He was told that shortly after arriving at the uncle's, she burst out laughing, said she had a stomachache, and then fell down unconscious. This scenario sounded implausible, and I told the father that something must be missing from his story, but I could draw no further information from him.

I inserted a tube through the girl's nose and with a hefty syringe started washing out her stomach. A beige-pink fluid studded with tiny pieces of feather and imbued with a fruity, fermented odor came up the tube. I was happy to point out to the father that unless the fish she had reportedly had for dinner had feathers, his accounting was clearly incomplete. He was unmoved. For that matter, there was no gumbo in the contents I was getting out of her stomach, and no fish either.

What exactly she had consumed I would never know, but our young patient was drunk and sunken in a deep alcoholic stupor. By the time the stomach pumping was finished, she had started to wake up, but for hours she was so wobbly and disoriented that I guessed she longed for a return of the coma.

Her father professed total ignorance as to how his daughter might have become inebriated, and I was powerless to insist on a credible explanation. We had to be satisfied that she would be well, at least for now.

6 April 2007

Good Friday

> At about 1:15 I went down to do a couple of ultrasounds when I passed one of my senior nurses shouting into his cell phone. I asked him if there was a problem. "That was my brother"—by which he meant fellow tribe member, not brother-brother—"in Gancé. Something is going on there. People are falling down. Seven. Then he said nine. He wanted the ambulance, but then a truck was passing by and they were coming in on that." Well, I said, we'll see them soon enough. I did my first ultrasound and had nearly finished the second when another nurse came down and said, "Docteur, we have an emergency."

> I went up to find a dozen bodies lying in different contortions on the sand behind my consulting room. Some were still, others were writhing, others were convulsing with generalized seizures. There were small children and young and middle-aged men and women. Shortly before falling ill, they had all eaten from

the same platter of millet and sauce. They were mostly field workers, and the boss's wife had fed them lunch, and the thinking was that maybe the millet had been contaminated by a pesticide.

I made a quick check of a few hearts and pupils and breaths and decided that if it were a pesticide, it wasn't the usual suspect, an organophosphate. That dismayed me momentarily, for at least we have an antidote to the organophosphate, and if it wasn't that, I didn't know what we might be dealing with. Then I saw some blood trickling from a few mouths, and once I ascertained that it didn't look like blood simply coming from bitten tongues of convulsing victims, I thought maybe it was rat poison (or rat poison mixed with something else?) that had been ingested.

I ordered injections of Vitamin K all around and we started getting nasogastric tubes down all these people. Only one NG tube was immediately available, so while someone went to dig the others out of a storeroom, I picked the two worst-looking men and started working on the one I thought was most far gone, pumping out the contents of his stomach. Within minutes the other tubes came and I got my best nurse working on the second fellow and one by one the other nurses working on the others.

Meanwhile more victims kept showing up, brought in by car or motorcycle, until there were 23 in all. It looked like a battlefield. Bodies writhing and seizing, babies crying, men shouting deliriously, toddlers clinging to their unconscious mothers, older children sitting in a daze, blood pouring from noses and mouths.

The nurses and all the rest of the staff performed magnificently, with calm discipline. Everyone was either assigned or assumed a role—putting down stomach tubes, pumping, dumping and fetching fresh buckets of water, carrying around trays of injections and syringes, preparing activated charcoal, holding down the convulsing and violently delirious patients, bringing gloves, opening packaging, controlling the crowd and chasing away the curious, eventually compiling a list of the victims. It seemed no more hectic or out of control than a cocktail party, the host pleasantly handing around trays of canapés and champagne.

We lost one man—the second of the two I had singled out at the beginning. Had I started with him and left the other, he would probably have lived and the other died—an eerie thought that sits uncomfortably in my brain. He died about 10 minutes into having his stomach pumped. The nurses who had been working on him crouched forlornly over his dead body. I told them to move on to the next person who needed help. The body lay flat on its back and a villager came and lifted the bottom of the man's t-shirt and folded it up to cover his face, a gesture of respect. There was no wailing for this death, no anguished ululating, so focused was everyone on the still living. The body lay there, just like that, the bottom of the shirt turned up over the face, through the whole raucous afternoon, and in the evening, when the storm had passed and the villagers lay exhausted but peacefully under our trees, his family asked permission to bury him. Granted.

We got home too late to care about dinner, but one of our diabetic patients who sat on the sidelines and watched the drama felt sorry for me and came over and gave me a loaf of sliced bread! This is a treat one rarely sees here. We took some pieces of cheese and sliced up a few of my old tomatoes that are almost dead but not quite, and I'll tell you that sandwich tasted better than a 5-star anything.

Where Things Get Done

Sunday, 22 April 2007

This is the heat we are having these days: 1) the butter—stick butter, not margarine—is liquid five minutes after it comes out of the fridge; 2) you can make a good cup of tea just by putting a tea bag in a cup of water that has been sitting on the counter; 3) without the benefit of a water heater, all showers are hot; 4) the DVD player (Canadian) shuts off every fifteen minutes; 5) ditto the projectors people try to use for PowerPoint presentations in meetings; 6) my camera smokes—smokes—when the flash goes off; 7) old men are being carried in wizened from dehydration; 8) the slightest illness in newborns causes their temperatures to shoot through the ceiling.

This morning I was called at 5 o'clock for a gunshot victim. The young man had been at home in his village when around midnight he was visited by thieves who shot him through the left eye. The eyeball was obliterated—no recognizable part of it remained—and the orbit was turned into hamburger laced with bone chips. We cleaned [the wound] and operated. The fellow is still alive tonight, but it is too early to know the extent of internal damage and whether he will live in the end. No bullet or shot was found, but I'm not sure this is a good thing. It might mean it passed through the side of his head, by the orbit, or it might mean it is lodged in his brain. If the latter, it makes little difference, for no one is going to try to go in and get it.

In June we broke ground for our new maternity and female medical ward. The bulk of the funding would be provided by Cimencam, Cameroon's main cement company, and in offering private corporate funding for a public establishment, it was an innovative venture for Cameroon. The building's completion would give us a place where women could deliver in a quiet, spacious environment, and moving out of the old maternity would free up much needed beds for sick patients. It would also allow us to finally house men and women in separate buildings.

Having enough beds and enough space was a constant problem, as was having enough time to do all that had to be done. The flow of outpatients was never ending, and getting them in and out was a daily challenge. Every tenth of a second counted.

Sometimes crises occurred simultaneously or in such quick succession that it was easy to lose track of them. As soon as I arrived at the hospital one Sunday morning, the two night nurses informed me that we had a woman fully dilated whose labor had been stalled since midnight. Worse, she was in her thirteenth pregnancy. We got the vacuum out and easily delivered an eleven-pound-nine-ounce girl. I left a nurse to look after the placenta and aftercare while I did my rounds and began the day's consultations.

My first patient was a man bent double in urinary retention. Next came a two-year-old comatose girl convulsing, and she was followed by a two-year-old boy, also convulsing. As I was treating him, the husband of the woman who had delivered the big baby came through my back door and said his wife seemed to be bleeding more than he thought she should. I jumped up and ran, knowing that women who bleed after their thirteenth child are likely to bleed a very great deal in a short time, and indeed she was pouring out blood. I sent the husband to collect three nurses. They came quickly, and we repositioned the woman to keep her brain perfused. While one of them started a drip through a thick needle in her arm, I reached in to rake the inside of her uterus. Our gloves cover only the hand and the wrist, so I was drenched to my elbow in blood as I reached and finally succeeded in snatching a strand of membrane that had been left behind. Once that was out, her bleeding stopped and the storm passed.

It had barely done so, though, and I had not finished what remained to be done when another nurse came into the delivery room to inform me that a delegation of people from the Ministry of Health in Yaoundé had arrived and were demanding to see me. They wanted to check the state of our vaccination program. I asked the nurse if she could handle them herself. She said she was willing, but they were in my office and would talk to no one but me.

I huffed, cursed under my breath, raged silently against our visitors for choosing a Sunday to come bother us, marched over to my office, held up my bloody arm so they would appreciate why I could not shake hands, and suggested that for now they see a nurse. Reluctantly, almost threateningly, I thought, they agreed.

I hated these bureaucrats with a passion I hid poorly. They were full of self-importance while being more ignorant and incapable than the lowliest nurse who actually had responsibility for patient care. As far as I could tell, they served little purpose beyond self-preservation and seemed oblivious to the fact that they were obstructing, often rudely, the real work of looking after those who needed what only we could provide.

After a while, once our critical patients were settled, I managed to sit with our visitors and give them all the information they sought. For years Kolofata had had the best vaccination coverage of any district in the country, but I suspected that a few months down the road when this delegation's report came out, rather than highlight our performance it would emphasize that on the day of their visit the ministry's delegation had been poorly received by an uncooperative doctor in charge who appeared to have little time or appreciation for their exalted selves.

As they were leaving, a wail ascended from the courtyard behind the female ward. I looked out and saw a crowd of women gathered. They were the women who had been attending the hospitalized wife of a local VIP. The couple had AIDS, and my first thought when I heard the wail was that the wife had died. I was not in the mood to deal with what was sure to be the resulting fiasco. I walked over with trepidation and was relieved to discover that she had not died, only fainted. We brought her round, and everyone settled back down.

Returning once again to my office, I received a text message from a Ministry of Health doctor in Yaoundé saying he needed a report now, if not before. This was a report I had already sent three times that Yaoundé had admitted repeatedly they had lost. I was fond of this particular doctor, so I hid my annoyance and sent the document yet again. But it occurred to me to wonder if Kolofata was the only place in the country where things got done.

Regarding health care, in any case. Electricity and water were increasingly off more often than they were on.

My Mother, I Am Dying

Tuesday, 10 July 2007

The evening ended with a Kolofata couple rushing into my room, the mother holding a flaccid one-year-old in her arms. The baby's eyes were idling back into her head, she was struggling for every breath, her conjunctivae and tongue were devoid of all color, and her liver and spleen were both engorged and dragging down towards her umbilicus—evidence that she had been sick for many days, if not weeks. I get beside myself in these cases. I do not understand how parents who live right down the road can let their children reach such a point before bringing them to hospital. They do not have a chance and neither do we. I ranted and raved and got the orders written up, but before we could even do the first test to match a donor, the child was dead. Cause of death: malaria-induced anemia. The anemia, or rather the severe anemia, she probably only had for a couple of days. The malaria she had surely had for a couple of weeks. To treat the malaria it would have cost the father less than a dollar. He would not spend that, or he was too preoccupied by other things, or he was out of town and the wife prohibited from going out without him, or who knows.

[A] premature baby on bed with us weighed in at 2 pounds [and was] named Alhere, which means luck. She is her [mother's] fourth child. The first three were also born prematurely and all died—not with us. When they brought this little

girl [she was] wrapped in cloth in a cardboard box and looked like a mouse in distress. The mother distanced herself from her and we had to work hard to get her to do what we asked. She kept saying there was no point, she knew what happens to babies like this, they only die. We told her that was certainly true, but this baby was not dead yet and she had to give her a fighting chance and maybe this time we would get lucky.

Sunday, 22 July 2007

A pair of teenaged boys crashed their motorcycle into a steel barrier. One of them has a head wound and a skull fracture and blood pouring out of his right ear and will not live, will not even regain consciousness. I see him lying there comatose on the bed and his mother sitting beside him and she has no idea, she just sees the outside scrapes and bruises and figures in a little while he will wake up and she will fix some porridge for him. But he will not wake up, and she has no idea, and that is almost unbearably excruciating to see.

Monday, 23rd. Alhere—lady Luck—went home today. She is beautiful.

On Saturday afternoon a motorcycle-driver, with a woman and three brown chickens as passengers, skidded and crashed into my Land Rover as I was heading up the hospital path. I did not see him until he was upon me and going down. I knew it was a man and a woman—the chickens I only saw afterwards—and I hoped there wasn't a baby tucked on the mother's back. The sound of the impact was a sickening one and I stopped and got out with a sickening feeling—what if a tire had run over a leg? What if the bike had crushed a baby?—and was washed with relief when I got around to the other side of the LR and found the two of them (no baby) upright and smiling sheepishly. Even the chickens were unperturbed. I brought the woman up to the hospital to check her out, and the man came up with his motorcycle, just to be sure there were no hidden injuries, but all was well. I was so happy. I have three lifelong phobias. One is being in a war, one is being kidnapped, and the third is being in an accident in which somebody dies.

Sunday, 12 August 2007

I told you about the two boys who were in a motorcycle accident and smashed themselves up. The one we patched up and he left after a week, but the other had blood and cerebral spinal fluid draining out of his right ear and was in a deep coma from the moment of impact. I was sure, positive, that he would never come out of that coma, and indeed he did not—until the fifteenth day, when he started to stir. And then by golly didn't he just go on all the way to waking up. Within a day or two he was walking with help and understanding what one said to him and soon enough he was eating on his own. And talking. Sort of. Singing his words is more what he started—and continues—to do. His words are slurred, but they are understandable, and his vocabulary and thoughts appear to be limited ("I want to go home now"), but they make sense. You can ask him a question ("What grade are you in at school?") and he will sing you the correct answer. I think his mother never doubted for a minute that he would come back to her. *I remember her sitting on the bed that first day, his head on her lap, just waiting for him to wake up. And then waiting and waiting and waiting. He is going to be a handful for a while now, but my guess is she is up to it.*

Sunday evening, 26 Aug. 2007

3½ year old Fanta was skinny and swollen and unconscious, and her mother, who held her in her arms, was crying and calling her name as if begging her not to leave. Fanta's breathing was already shallow and irregular. Her hair was sparse, her feet swollen, her chest all jutting ribs—typical severe malnutrition. When the mother brought her into my consulting room I had to look carefully to see that Fanta was still alive, so still and dead did she look. With nothing to lose, I filled a syringe with 50% dextrose—sugar—found a vein and pushed it in. Within a few minutes her eyes were open and she was looking about and finally responded when her mother called her name. She has a long road yet ahead, but that was a nice first step. She was literally starving to death and was minutes if not seconds from getting there.

Saturday, 01 September 2007

The adolescent boy with the caved in skull who was in coma and who when he woke up at last could only sing his speech—he came back for a follow-up visit last week and had us all agog. But for the dent in the side of the head, which lends him a bit of panache, he appears to be perfect. He talks, no longer sings, and although he has no recollection of what happened to him and has been in no hurry to get back on a motorcycle, he seems to know everything he is supposed to know, walks and talks normally, plans to show up for school like all his comrades this Monday.

One Friday morning in early September I finished my rounds by six o'clock and set out with Myra for a meeting in Maroua. We had had a big rain the day before, and there were rumors of flooding in several villages, so I wasn't sure how far we would get or how hard it would be to get there, but once we crossed our first causeway with little difficulty, I began to relax. As we approached the second causeway, that insouciance changed.

The river was running high and the current fast. It had already overflowed its banks and flooded fields for hundreds of meters around. The road itself leading up to the bridge was eroded. A crowd of thirty or forty people stood at each edge, staring at the rushing water and at the abyss that had to be jumped to get even to the causeway, let alone to the other side. We talked with them and learned about the villages that had been flooded. They told us that water ran chest-high through the middle of some of them. Mud houses had dissolved. Granaries full of millet had burst open and washed away. Canvas sacks of millet had sunk. In some villages every home had been destroyed, and families had lost everything they owned. To keep from drowning, children had had to be hoisted onto backs and shoulders, where they stayed through the night. The only people who had slept were those who could rescue a soggy mat or mattress and set it in a tree or on undissolved bricks piled high enough to poke out of the water.

Unable to go farther or to be of assistance in the moment, we turned back. We concocted an illustrated pamphlet to warn people of postflood dangers: (1) Don't drink the flood water. (2) Use mosquito nets. (3) Stay out of damaged houses and away from cracked walls that might crumble without warning. (4) Don't try to cross rivers with roaring currents. (5) Keep your children away from the river edge and know where they are at all times. We multiplied these and started finding ways to distribute them to affected villages, and we used the rest of the day to go out to whatever villages we could reach, talking to people and phoning others to get the most information we could about the extent of the flooding and the damage.

By the end of the day we had a good idea of the situation, and I phoned Amadou Ali to see if there was anything he might do to help. At first he was simply angry that the local authorities were showing little interest or initiative, but when I explained to him that apart from the other health hazards, I was afraid that within a week people would be going hungry, he calmed down and said yes, he could help. He told me who to see to access his warehouse and who else to see to get cash, and he instructed me to distribute sacks of millet and envelopes of cash to the people most hurt by the floods. He asked me to make it clear to the people that government aid would come later. For now this was a personal contribution. I was to be sure none of it fell into the hands of our local authorities, whence it stood too good a chance of disappearing.

We followed his instructions to the letter and spent the weekend and through the following Tuesday distributing millet and money to tide people over until the government could organize more substantial relief. Villagers worked tirelessly and ingeniously to cobble together shelters from pieces of wood, metal, and other materials salvaged from the flood, sleeping at night in schools, mosques, and rickety lean-tos.

In time the villages were rebuilt, all but one in the same place, with structures no more solid and no grander than before.

Monday, 19 November 2007

> *As I was rounding the corner to visit the last two rooms of the isolation ward during my evening rounds yesterday, I heard a man groaning and a woman sobbing. The wrenching sounds seemed to be coming from Djoro's room, and I feared the worst. Djoro is a young man of about 25 from a village only 12 km from Kolofata. In 2006 he was found to have tuberculosis and put on a 6-month course of treatment that he abandoned after the first 2 months because the medicines made him feel queasy.*
>
> *Someone with TB is better never to go on treatment than to go on and stop partway, but getting patients to understand and accept this is difficult and we*

do not always succeed. Djoro could not be coaxed back until the sickness was again so bad he could hardly walk. The problem with defaulters is that their lungs suffer that much more scarring and their germ becomes resistant to our drugs. Chronic ear infections through childhood had left Djoro mostly deaf, so he had that to cope with as well. His mother, a robust grey-haired motherly woman, cared for him round the clock, though he often could be cruelly dismissive of her ministrations. He has been deteriorating for the past few weeks and no combination of medicines seemed to touch him. One evening last week his mother came running into my room crying that he was dying. I went back with her and he wasn't, not then anyway, though he had been vomiting all day and was dehydrated and weak.

I went into their room and Djoro was lying on his bed moaning eerily and his mother was sitting beside him, wringing her hands and weeping, My son, my son. Djoro's limbs are just sticks and his thorax is all ribs and the skin on his face is stretched over the bones of his skull like a mummy's. I called to him—he is deaf but he can hear if you stand in front of him and shout—and he stopped moaning and looked at me. I am dying, he said. His mother sobbed. He looked at her and reached out to touch her and said, My mother, I am dying, and then puddles of tears filled his eyes too and the two of them cried together, though you could see him trying not to. Then he looked again at me and explained, Death has found me; death finds everyone, doesn't it, and now it has found me, and if I die, I die, isn't that right? Yes, I said, but Djoro, you are not going to die right now. He was breathless and his voice was hoarse and I was amazed at his coherence. But wait, he said, wait: I want to go home. Tomorrow, I said; now night is coming; but tomorrow. I can go home tomorrow? he asked. If you want, I said. Then listen, he said. Death has found me, but death finds everyone, so death has found me, and if I die tonight, then I die and that is okay, but if I don't die, then tomorrow I go home, is that right? That's right, I said, that's right. And he went over it again and then again, to be sure.

He lived through the night and this morning said he was feeling a little better. But he weakened as the day wore on, and when his brother showed up this afternoon to take him home, Djoro slipped into a coma, at peace at last.

I'm Going to Carry You on My Back

A SCHOOLBOY WENT out to the roofless latrine behind his primary school to relieve himself one Thursday morning in February. He undid the drawstring of his trousers and looked down into the pit, which was not as deep as it should have been. The sun evidently was at just the right angle in the sky, for when the boy looked down he had no doubt that what he saw below was a baby lying belly-up.

He decided he could hold whatever he had intended to excrete, did up his pants, and shot out of the latrine like an arrow off a bow. He went straight to his principal, who went straight to the commandant of Kolofata's gendarmerie, who came straight to me.

One of my pet peeves was the preference of people to eschew latrines in favor of nature when nature called, but on this day I was happy the latrine had been so little used. Looking down the hole, it was clear the baby was not alive. She didn't move, and even from on high one foot looked to be on the greener side of the spectrum. We brainstormed for a quarter of an hour trying to decide what might be the best way of getting the body out, but eventually some iron rebar and a rope with a slipknot did the job.

She was a beautiful full-term baby, or at least she had been, at one time, beautiful. A surgical mask did nothing to block the putrid odor, and to examine her I had to compete with hundreds of sticky, stubborn, furious flies. The left side of her thorax and abdomen were swamp-water green, and her skin sloughed off in sheets. Tiny ants had gnawed tiny holes in her right cheek and right forearm. The severed umbilical cord was dried, beige and untied. Rigor mortis had worn off, and so she was as soft and supple as a living newborn, and but for the fact that she was dead and rotting, she was perfect in every way.

The gendarmes and police often attributed unrealistic powers to medical professionals. We were not pathologists, we had no coroners to consult, and the autopsies we did were superficial examinations. Calling this a case of infanticide (though there was no evidence the baby had died after birth as opposed to before), the commandant wanted me to say how and when she had perished and who had done what to her. I could offer with some degree of certainty a vague "when," and since there was no bruising or bleeding, it seemed likely that she had died before being tossed into the latrine, but for more answers than these, I could be of no help.

The dutiful gendarmes were angry at the unknown alleged perpetrator and, craving justice, were unsatisfied with my report. I was only sad, suffused with grief for the lost mother and for the baby she had—or someone had—thrown away.

Monday, 07 April 2008

> *My desk is top-heavy with paperwork. We are up to over 60 monthly reports now—each one up to 10 pages long—and there is the vaccination campaign report, another fifty pages all in triplicate, and there is the next chapter of reports compiled for the Ministry's 5-year (actually 4-year now because they got started late) plan and that is spiral-bound in 8 separate volumes, each one between 30 and 60 pages long, plus there are a handful of file folders containing multiple page reports of this and that, most waiting to be wrapped up, photocopied and spiral-bound. No one can possibly have any use for all this stuff. No one can*

possibly read through it all. No one can possibly want to. It is pure scandal, the time and energy and forests consumed by this drudgery. I have upped my order to 100 reams of paper this year. 50,000 sheets. Myra says she doubts it will be enough, and she might be right. The government requires all this busywork, but it is only the government in that aid agencies (WHO, The Global Fund, UNCEF, etc.) work through the government and it is the aid agencies that want it. I think they haven't got a clue the extent to which their bureaucratic demands drain human, material and financial resources at the grass roots where those things are so precious and rare.

All this documentation does not stop the corruption. In a way it worsens it, for now the government-employed thieves all along the hierarchical chain simply produce bills and reports (faked) to prove they have not stolen. It is a racket and many people are making a fine living off these programs. And meanwhile the AIDS medicines run out, the mosquito nets disappear, the reagents for testing for TB and HIV never make it up-country. But on we go, writing our hundreds and hundreds and hundreds of pages of reports. In triplicate, spiral-bound.

Monday, 26 May 2008

We have a 70 year old lady on bed with us. Ramata. I first met her when she was slumped outside my office door late one afternoon, devoting all the energy she had to being able to breathe. White disheveled hair, puffy eyelids, sagging layers of cheek, eyes blinded by cataracts, swollen hands and feet, infected wounds on her right thumb oozing pus. The family had to carry her into my office and eventually to the ward, and over the next two weeks we set about treating her multiple problems—getting her heart failure under control, cleaning up the infection, and removing one of the cataracts. From the moment she started getting better, she was beside herself with glee. "As soon as I can walk again," she said to me every morning on rounds, "I'm going to carry you on my back." And when she was able to walk again—and see again, too—every morning it was, "Come on," tapping her back, "let me wrap you on my back," and the nurses and her fellow patients would giggle and slap each other's hands. She will go home today or tomorrow.

Sunday, 26 October 2008

Yesterday started off with a woman referred from a health center outside our district. We've been getting more and more of these, and I guess it's all right, but I also wish their own hospitals worked better so they could take care of themselves. The nurse had written in the referral note, "Fearful for the life of his wife and child, the patient's husband wants to go see the doctor in Kolofata." (Everyone, even out there, knows the doctor in Kolofata by name, and at one point as I was assessing the patient, a woman in her party walked in and said to the nurse beside me, "Is that Elène?" "Yes," replied the nurse. "Aha!" rejoined the lady, putting a hand to her mouth. My guess is she expected someone a little—I don't know; taller, thicker, more imposing.) It was a first pregnancy for the patient, and she had been in labor for 3 days. Her water had been broken for two of them. She was fully dilated and the head was well down, but it had been so squeezed by the narrow birth canal that it had taken the shape of a zucchini. We dug out the vacuum that had been gathering dust since June. The baby, a girl, came out flat and purple as a blueberry pancake, but she had just enough of a heartbeat to give us hope. So we went to work on her for the next hour, and just when it looked like we might lose her after all, she practically sprang to life. Started breathing on her own, moving her legs, her arms, even emitted a whimper. By the time we handed her to her mother, she was ready to suck.

Sunday, 2 Nov. My birthday baby [the blueberry pancake baby, born on my birthday] should be discharged tomorrow. I have felt happy all week because of her. Maybe, 54 years ago, I was born for no other reason but to allow her to be born and live.

Obama City

Friday, 7 November 2008

I got to bed late Tuesday night and got up early—2 AM—Wednesday morning in order to follow CNN's coverage of the election returns. Knowing it would be exciting and historic, I did not want to spend the rest of my life regretting having missed the blow-by-blow. So I followed it all, at times sitting in my chair, at times lying on the rug on the floor, bundled in a couple of small tablecloths to ward off the nighttime chill. CNN did an excellent job, and I watched riveted. I almost felt I was there, in the hotels, on the streets, in the studio, at Grant Park in Chicago.

It is difficult to describe the elation we have encountered here. I have been receiving telephone calls, text messages, notes and comments of congratulations all week—not something that has happened after any previous election. Our nurses Wednesday morning were honking their motorcycle horns, dancing and singing "Obama, Obama" and "We can do it!"—They didn't quite get the "Yes, we can," but I like their version just as much. While it is understandable that Africans would like to see an African American elected president of the United States, this unrestrained ebullience took me by surprise.

AA was one of the callers this week. "Docteur, congratulations on your revolution!" he said right away. "Revolution?" I asked. "Well, not for you, not for America, but for the rest of the world, this is a revolution, and a very good thing." He went on to say: of course, the white man is very sly and perhaps he has set up this black man to fail. I said maybe, but probably he was our best bet not to fail. With that he agreed and predicted that practically overnight the world's ill will (hatred is the word he used) toward the U.S. would dissipate. I talked a little about how high expectations had been drawn and that disappointment was inevitable. He replied that he thought disappointment was inevitable only among black Americans who perhaps thought a black president would cater to them, and Obama to his mind did not seem like the kind of person who would be doing that. ("And by the way, he picked as his chief of staff a Jew! A Jew! And now they are going to solve the Israel-Palestine problem!" he added.) I told him I wore an American flag pin on Wednesday—just for the one day, something I have never done before. "You were right to do that," he said. "Today every American has the right to be proud."

So now we have to keep this man safe, and failing to do so would be a calamity that would trump the triumph of this week a thousand times over.

Saturday, 29 November 2008

I was called at midnight on—Monday, I think it was, maybe Tuesday—for a woman in obstructed labor. Her fourth child, and she had been in labor for five days. She was in considerable distress. Her abdomen was huge and looked huger because it was swollen with subcutaneous fluid. In fact her whole perineum, including the labia, as well as the thighs, legs and feet were swollen with retained fluid. She was not anemic and she had a normal blood pressure—two things which, if abnormal, might have given us a clue as to what was going on. We could not hear a fetal heart. She was dilated only about 5 cm. Before I got there the nurses had informed the family that she would be going for surgery, and they (the family) were heartsick at the thought. I went to the ultrasound room and lugged our clunky ultrasound over to the delivery room. Putting the probe on the mother's mountainous abdomen, I found the baby—alive!—pressed back almost against the mother's spine. What was pressing it back was fluid that absolutely filled the abdomen, from the pelvis to the chest. But it wasn't free fluid in the abdomen and it wasn't amniotic fluid. It seemed to be separated from the baby by a thin membrane. Oh my goodness, I said to myself, and to the nurse I said, let's catheterize her. And so we did, and over the next ten minutes a good 5 or 6 liters of urine came flowing happily out. The sumo belly deflated. The baby no doubt felt a huge weight lifted from his tiny shoulders. The mother-to-be fell asleep. The nurse kept saying ooh and aah. I went home and back to bed. In the morning, just as we got to her on rounds, the woman delivered. A lively boy. I kept the catheter in for a couple of days to give her bladder a rest, but then I took it out to see if she could urinate and empty the bladder. She could and she did, and yesterday they went home.

I never knew that a bladder could hold that much urine, but now I do, so next time I feel like I just have to go, I'll know it's not true.

When we were in Maroua last week, we noticed a water tap on the side of a squiggly little road leading into the city. Most people, even in the city, do not have running water. They get their water from wells or pumps or the river, or sometimes [from] these roadside taps that are rented by someone who sits there all day and for a few francs allows people to come and fill their buckets. This tap was being rented by a teenaged boy, and he had constructed a tin roof over it to give him shade, and what made us notice it was that at the edge of the road

he had put up a sign whose letters, painted in whitewash, said, OBAMA CITY,
with an arrow underneath pointing toward the tap. I asked Minista, our driver,
to stop and I got out and asked who was the chief of this place, and the boy
stepped forward. I said I liked his sign and could I take a picture of it. Of course,
he said. I asked him if he'd like to be in the picture, and he said sure, why not,
and so he posed. I thanked him, and as I was getting back into the car he said,
"Obama—tell him to think about us." I told him yes I would, next time I see him.

The Canadian High Commission encouraged us to apply for a grant for the construction of our next building, which would be a women's pavilion dedicated primarily to antenatal care and education. Canadian law required that funds destined for construction could be conferred only upon submission of a report by an appropriate expert attesting to the impact the construction would likely have on the environment. The Ministry of the Environment had trained people whose job was to do this work, and we were told that any group requesting their services was responsible only for getting them to and from the site of the proposed construction.

Myra and I went to Maroua one day to talk to the head of the province's Environment Ministry. We showed him the plan of the building and explained what was needed. He declared that since the building was relatively small and on the inside of a walled-off compound, the request was ridiculous, and all I needed was a declaration signed by his office stating as much. It could be done, he assured us, in a flash. He then introduced us to François, his assistant, and asked us to work out the details with him.

We followed François into a bare little room and showed him our papers and explained our request, and after some lighthearted muttering and dithering he disappeared from the room. He came back two minutes later and stated his price, which was $1,200. I squinted back at him, wondering if I had heard him correctly. He assured me that I had. I told him that we did not have that kind of money. We thanked him, gathered up our papers, and left.

Driving back to Kolofata, we considered our options, which were few. We thought about tapping a man in Mora or another in Kolofata. The former was also with the Environment Ministry but lower down the ladder, and the latter was with the Forest Ministry, which perhaps was close enough to pass muster. The problem with both choices was that the men were sufficiently uneducated that we would probably have to write the report ourselves and ask them to sign it, which did not seem to be in the spirit of the Canadian concern.

We were just outside Mora and still mulling this over when we got a phone call. It was the $1,200 man from Maroua. I guessed that François or his boss had done some asking around after we left, found out who we were, and discovered that ours was the village of the minister of justice, who as it happened was in the process of hauling the more corrupt of the highs and mighties before the courts. I could hear the panic in his voice.

"I can come," he said. "Right now, this very minute, if you'd like. Just say the word."

"We can't afford you," I replied.

"No, no," he insisted, "it will not cost anything. Nothing at all. I will bring my own computer, my own printer. Don't worry about a thing. I don't want anything from you, not one franc. I can come right now if you want."

I smiled, gave Myra a thumbs-up. "Monday would be fine. I'll be waiting for you at the hospital at seven thirty."

Monday he came closer to seven thirty than I had expected. He brought his own computer, his own printer, his own paper, and his own secretary, and he stayed for two days. By the time he left we had our report, signed, sealed, stamped, and delivered. We gave him two hundred dollars and a thank-you, and for this he seemed surprised, grateful, and relieved.

Saturday, 27 December 2008

Last Sunday we received the governor of Borno State, Nigeria, for an official visit to the hospital. He is governor of a relatively wealthy state in one of Africa's wealthiest, most powerful, and they would say most sophisticated countries. Borno State has a well-developed capital city and a network of teaching hospitals throughout. I've seen patient files from those hospitals: they have fancy laboratories, imaging departments and every specialty imaginable. And yet the people come to Kolofata for health care, braving the long trip, the border crossing, the foreign police, the strange language and money. I think he expected to find a colossal multistory gleaming technologically buzzing ultramodern and ultra comfortable institution bursting with equipment, brimming with doctors. And instead he found what we are: a bush hospital. He asked how many patients we see a day and I said about a hundred and he asked how many Nigerians and I said about half, and he only nodded sadly. He never asked me why I thought they came here and I don't know what conclusions he drew himself.

If You Shake Their Hands, Your Testicles Fall Off

MAGIC COURSED THROUGH Kolofata like blood through a body. It was ever-present and essential to life. One did not talk of believing in it or not believing in it: it was just *there*, everywhere, in everything, every event, and everyone knew it. I was expected to know it as well.

A young shepherd tending his flock was attacked, bludgeoned, stabbed, and left for dead as the thug and a younger brother made off with his sheep. When the shepherd did not come home that evening, his father went looking for him, found him in a field, prostrate but still alive, and carried him to hospital. His injuries were serious but not beyond repair. Once fixed up and discharged, he filed suit against his attacker, whom he had recognized. As required by law, I submitted a medical certificate detailing the shepherd's injuries.

The father of the thief, a well-known livestock rustler, learned that his boy was about to be arrested, so he decided to countersue, claiming that it was the shepherd who had attacked his son. Therefore the son, too, would need a medical certificate to present to the judge to support his accusation, so the father brought the youth to me and proceeded to describe with much disdain and vigor how his son had been attacked and brutally stabbed by the perfidious shepherd. The father walked over to his boy.

"Here." He pointed to his son's sternum. "And here." He pointed to the right shoulder. "And here." He pointed to his neck.

"Yes," I said, "well, let's see," and I asked the young man to remove his tunic. Try as I might to imagine some small nick, bruise, or swelling, I saw nothing.

"I see nothing," I said.

"Oh no," the father replied, "you won't see it." He produced from the folds of his own tunic a ten-inch dagger that had been bent into a perfect semicircle. "My boy is protected by a spell. A knife cannot harm him." He held the dagger out for me to inspect. "See what happened when they tried to stab him?" he rejoiced. "Don't you see? Here is where he was stabbed"—he pointed to his son's chest— "and here is the knife. Ha! *Here*," he repeated, marveling, holding up with a certain reverence the semicircular blade, "is the knife!"

I studied the father, looked at the knife, looked at the boy whose eyes remained downcast.

"Aha," I said, "there is the knife!" and I dutifully filled out the medical certificate, citing evidence of neither injury nor magical spell and omitting all mention of mystically curved daggers.

The boy was arrested and locked up, and I subsequently heard that the father paid—he did, after all, have spare sheep to sell—to get him out before he had to stand trial.

Wednesday, 14 January 2009

We gathered as usual outside the male ward before morning rounds yesterday morning. This is a daily 5-minute mini-meeting where we go over things that happened in the night and anticipate things expected for the day ahead. People will also sometimes make announcements at this gathering—about a birth in the family or an illness or theft they heard about in town. Yesterday, after the off-going night nurses gave report and we were set to break up to begin rounds, one of our senior and most highly trained nurses spoke up. "There is magic going on in Maroua." What do you mean? I asked. "There are people going around shaking hands, and if you shake the hand of one of these people, your testicles fall off." Oh my, I said, feeling Fabien's (our [French] med student's) eyes popping out behind me. Most of the other nurses were aware of this calamity. "They have already made two arrests, two men are in jail for it," offered one. "It's said that somewhere in Maroua there is a whole room filled with piled up testicles," offered another. "It is spreading to Mora," offered a third. This was getting close to home. Everyone turned to Kakiang who lives in Mora and commutes each day. "Is that true, Kakiang?" Yes, he said, he had heard that it was, but so far he had not seen it happen with his own eyes. Another nurse told of a friend of a friend it had happened to, in a town outside Maroua. Everyone shivered and agreed it would be wise not to shake hands with strangers for a while. I told our consultant nurses to be on the lookout for castrated men and let me know if any came in. And then we started our rounds.

Tuesday, 24 March 2009

This afternoon I get a call from my head nurse in Amchide, up at the border. "Doctor," he says, "I have a situation." This is what he says when he is having a problem out of the ordinary. I tense as I always do when I hear Pascal say he has a situation. "What's up?" I say. "I have two men here," he replies, "who are saying that someone has snatched their penises." I am in the middle of rounds in the male ward. Fabien is beside me. I repeat, "Someone has snatched their penises?" Fabien stops in his tracks, startled, tenser now than I. "Yes," Pascal says. "That's what they say." "Well, and what do you find when you examine them?" "Everything is there," Pascal says, "right where you'd expect it to be." "Okay, well I guess that's good. Did you ask them what exactly they mean when they say someone snatched their penises?" He had asked them and the only thing he'd managed to get out of one of them was that he could no longer have an erection. "Since when?" I ask. "Since this morning," Pascal says. Seems a little premature for these guys to start panicking and I tell Pascal just to handle it and I ask him if there is some problem from his point of view that he is not telling me about. "No no," he says, "but the police are here and they are going to need a report." Ah ha. This is the crux. I am the only one who can write an official medical report. As much as anything else, he is warning me. I thank him, tell him to do the complete physical, write it up and send it to me so I'll have it when the police make their formal request. Apparently there will be an investigation into these penis-snatchings-that-aren't and I'll bet you someone will be arrested and sent to prison.

Saturday, 28 March. [Let me] jot down the latest chapter. Friday morning at 2:00 I was called because two badly beaten up men had been brought in with multiple stab wounds and contusions. Here is the story we got from the gendarmes who accompanied them. The two men were from a village near Mora. They had gone home to their ancestral village southwest of Kolofata to attend the funeral of an uncle. Coming back Thursday night by motorcycle, they stopped at our village of Talkomari, about 10 km from Kolofata, to get gas. They filled up, paid, and then took off, and at that moment the gas seller realized that he had suddenly lost his genitals. He started shouting, rousing the town, telling them to stop the genital thieves, SOS, SOS, SOS. The town, and the next town, [took] off after these guys, caught them, confiscated their motorcycles, and set about beating them with sticks and machetes. By a quirk of good fortune, a gendarme was in the town—it had been market day, and to minimize the dangers of the inevitable market day drunkenness the gendarmes generally post an officer in the town on market day. He was able to get the mob off the men and save their lives. We patched them up and they spent the rest of the night in the police station for their own protection.

In the morning, the gas seller showed up at the hospital and bought ($3.00) a medico-legal report form. He took a number, and when it was his turn he entered my consulting room, sat down, and when asked what his problem was replied that two men had stolen his genitals in the night and he wanted me to fill out the medico-legal report so he could take it as proof to the police. What exactly happened? I asked. He explained that these two strangers had stopped at his gas stand the night before, filled their motorcycles and paid, and in the instant that they started their engines and took off, he felt a shock, like a burst of cold, shoot through his body and he realized that these guys had stolen his genitals. Why don't you show me what you mean, I suggested, and he was happy I asked and unbuckled his belt right away and unzipped his pants and reached in and pulled out in his fist . . . a perfectly fine penis and two testicles snug in their sac, everything attached and in its rightful place. I said to him, it looks like everything is there. But look, he said, can't you see, the penis is shrunken, and my testicles hurt. The testicles were of normal size, shape and form, as was the penis. I asked him about pain or blood on urination, discharge and so on and he reported no complaints on any count. I asked what happened to the strangers and he said the townsmen beat them up. I asked if the pain in his testicles was worse or better now than it had been in the night. He said a little better. Actually, he explained, as soon as those men were caught and beaten up, the pain started to go down. I filled out the report, duly making note of the everything that was there and the nothing that was not, signed it, stamped it with my three different official stamps, two black and one green, STAMP STAMP STAMP, and handed the paper to him. He took it and trotted off to the police station.

As we were shooting the breeze before rounds that day, a nurse volunteered that he knew of a case of genital theft that happened in Maroua. The victim went to the police and the police sent him to the hospital for medical assessment. The doctor examined him, found everything in place and in order and told the guy so. "But," the man said, "this is not my penis. This one belongs to someone else. They took mine." "Look," he said, "see those pimples? My penis doesn't have pimples." The doctor called in the guy's wife to corroborate, and this she did. "That," she declared, looking at the disputed organ, "is not my husband's penis. My husband's penis does not have pimples." The nurse could not tell us what happened after that, but this problem is causing considerable unrest throughout the province.

Aren't you glad you live in a country where by and large the only thing pickpockets pick is pockets?

Saturday, 31 October 2009

A woman came to me the other day armed with a medico-legal report form. She was about 50 years old, married, had never had children. [Her] complaint was that she had repeatedly been accused of being a witch and since she was not a witch she was sick and tired of being thus accused and to put an end to the rumors and insults and accusations—and stick throwing, apparently—she wanted me the doctor to set down in writing that she was not a witch. She had scraped together several weeks' worth of income to buy the form, and she was willing to undergo whatever tests I felt necessary to prove that she was not a witch. I listened intently and proceeded to examine her head to toe using all my gadgets—the BP cuff with its needle gauge, the thermometer with its beep, the oximeter with its red LED lights—and in the end solemnly announced (and wrote on the form) that after a thorough examination I found no evidence whatsoever of her being a witch. I further wrote on the form that she was in grave physical and emotional danger of suffering significant incapacity, should anyone accuse her of being a witch. I signed the form, stamped it, and told her to take it to the police.

Today a similar case occurred. I was at home on break when a policeman brought a pair of co-wives to the hospital. Calvin, the nurse on duty, told me afterwards what happened. The second wife was accusing the first wife of being a witch, of having eaten her daughter-in-law. The first wife denied she was a witch and said she had nothing to do with her daughter-in-law's untimely death. Rather than duke it out, the two of them went to the police to settle the matter. The police chief, at a loss, brought them to hospital. The second wife told Calvin she wanted the first wife checked out by whatever machines we had to prove she was a witch. Calvin listened. He asked the first wife if she agreed to be tested. The first wife said she was not a witch, she didn't even know what a witch was or how a witch ate people, and she had nothing to fear. Okay, Calvin said, sit there. She sat. He got out the sphygmomanometer and held it up. "I'm going to put this around your arm." She agreed. "Now are you sure you're not a witch? Because if you are, when I start pressing this bulb, it will cause you to faint right away and you may never be able to get up." The second wife, watching, nodded in approval and cheered him on, "Unhuhn, unhuhn." The first wife told him to go ahead. And so he did, pumped the thing up to 220 mmHg—and the lady did not fall. He released the pressure. The second wife expressed surprise, disbelief. "Wait a minute," Calvin said, "we're not finished." He got out his mercury thermometer and held it up. "I'm going to put this under your arm," he said. "Now are you sure you're not a witch? Because if you are, when I put this under your arm, you are going to pop up out of your chair. We've had people pop so high and hard they go right through the ceiling." The second wife nodded with satisfaction. "Unhuhn, unhuhn." The first wife remained unfazed and lifted her arm. The temperature was taken, and she did not take off. Calvin waited a respectable time, waited, waited. Nothing. "Well," he said to the first wife and the second wife and the policeman, "that's as good a proof as you'll find anywhere. This lady is not a witch." The policeman and the first wife thanked him, and even the second wife accepted his verdict, and off they all went.

Here, Take This, Please, Fix It

14 November 2010

*A few days ago, in the afternoon just as the hospital was shutting down and the bulk of the staff were packing up to leave, a Kolofata woman burst into my consulting room. She was shouting, but hoarsely—she couldn't get her breath—and her eyes were wide and wild. A three year old dead-looking body was draped in her arms, and this she held out to me, as they do ("*HERE—TAKE THIS—PLEASE—FIX IT—FIX IT*") and I could see right away that the girl wasn't breathing. I didn't bother to check if she was dead or alive but assumed or hoped it was the latter, since there was no sense assuming she was dead, and rushed her down to the delivery room, the only place, apart from surgery, where we have oxygen. A couple of nurses and Anne our [Australian] medical student were with me, and we started working on the girl—who was not, as it turned out, dead, but who would not, would* NOT, *breathe. All the while the mother was intermittently pacing the floor and throwing herself down onto it, rolling around in barely contained rage and grief and muttering things about the husband, how he was sitting at home doing nothing, how he had seen the state of his daughter and done nothing, how he was lazy and mean and good for nothing. The girl had convulsed and saliva had clogged her throat, blocking her airway, and in her postictal state she hadn't the strength or the consciousness to unblock it. Suctioning her throat got her to take a couple of breaths, but she had been unbreathing for long enough that her brain was depressed and she was little inclined to take more than those first breaths. We stayed on her for forty-five minutes before she started breathing on her own. She remained unconscious, though, so I told Anne to stay with her and suction her occasionally while I went back to my office for half an hour to tend to other things.*

Fifteen minutes later Anne came to say the girl was not doing well, was seizing again. I went back down, stopped the seizure, settled her down, left her once more in the care of Anne and a nurse, and returned to my office. The seizure was frightening but everything else indicated that she was doing better so I was not much worried.

Ten minutes later the distraught mother threw herself into my office and wailed again about the rotten husband and said she wanted to take her daughter home. She remembered now, she said, that the night before a dog had barked furiously outside their compound, and that could not have been for nothing: a spell had been cast and she must get her daughter to a marabout. And furthermore the rotten husband said he was not coming and was not going to pay a single franc for any care his daughter might be getting at the hospital. I know the rotten husband—who is indeed rotten but not poor; he has a job and a salary—and in fact the wife, the woman before me now, had had an ectopic pregnancy in August and we had saved her life and he still had a major bill outstanding for that. I listened to this, and nodded in sympathy to the bit about the dog, and then told her sternly that that child was going nowhere, not home and not to a marabout, and the rotten husband was to get his rotten bones up here and in front of me right here right now.

Ten minutes later he did that and then it was his turn to rant about the dog and about how his child had been seized by the devil and was dying and anyone could see that and he for my information was not going to pay one franc not one franc. Wrong on all counts, I told him, and go comfort your wife.

Over the course of the evening the seizures stopped, the fever subsided, and we got her off oxygen. By morning she was sitting up drinking porridge, her mother next to her and beside herself as much as she had been the day before, but this time with gratitude. The rotten husband quietly paid up, every last franc, and the next day they all went home, a happy little family.

Among the joys of working in a resource-poor subtropical environment were the frequency and relative simplicity with which we could relieve suffering and save lives. One of the conditions we had little hope of curing, though, was cancer, and of all the cancers, the ones that hit children were the most heart wrenching.

Retinoblastoma is a tumor of the eye that occurs especially in children under the age of five years throughout the world. Untreated in time, it is invariably fatal. In industrialized countries, parents notice a yellowish discoloration of the pupil and bring the child to the doctor. In rural Africa, parents notice a yellowish discoloration of the pupil and figure there are worse things in life. So they do nothing. The tumor grows; it destroys the eyeball, starts to overflow the socket, and finally at some point the parent starts to take notice and wonder why the eye is looking like that. They carry the child to a health center where chances are the nurse, who has never heard of retinoblastoma, thinks the condition is just an unusual infection and treats it with a topical ointment that turns out to be useless. So they take him to the local healer who does his magic with red-legged chickens, porcupine quills, cat claws, or whatever, and that turns out to be useless as well. But while these useless treatments are being tried, one after the other, the tumor is growing, and it is growing in three dimensions at once.

Often not until the tumor was the size of a golf ball or even a tennis ball would the family eventually make its way to us. We had no top-of-the line antineoplastic agents, no cryotherapy or radiotherapy. We could offer palliative surgery, but it was only a pitiable prelude to inevitable death. More often we simply shook our heads, explained our regret, and sent these children away.

Ophthalmo Sans Frontières, or OSF, the French NGO that energetically spearheaded and supported our ophthalmology service, became interested in seeing whether more could be done. They obtained for us a limited selection of relatively inexpensive antineoplastic agents and consulted with experts to help us develop a medicosurgical protocol for managing children suffering from retinoblastoma. Patients underwent two cycles of preoperative chemotherapy, then surgical removal of the eye, and finally two cycles of postoperative chemotherapy. The regime was brutal and many of our young charges still died, but there were also enough early successes to encourage us to continue.

12 February 2011

One of [our retinoblastoma patients] right now is a 3 year old named Adèle, a girl from the other side of the country, by Chad. Like many of these children, she was miserable when she first came. The cancerous eye was a lime-sized tumor that hung out of her head, dripping pus. She screamed—screamed—whenever anyone came near her. Her mother was the epitome of patience, even when Adèle in her anger and frustration lashed out wildly at her with her little fists. I made it my goal to get her to smile. This was quite a job, made worse by the fact that we were constantly prodding her, sticking her, taking blood from her. I went to see her every morning and every evening—the screaming started as soon as she saw me approach. Sometimes I would talk softly to her right through her screams, sometimes I would make a point of talking only to her mother. Sometimes I would examine her, sometimes I would not touch her at all. It was slow going, but after a couple of weeks the screaming stopped. Then one day she extended her hand when I reached out to shake. And then [another] day she was sitting on the floor eating from a bowl of rice when I came over to see her and without flinching she reached into her rice, found a nice big piece of fish meat, and held it out to me. I took it, thanked her, gave it back. The next day she had a cookie for me. And a couple of days ago she and her mother were up in the waiting room when I came into the building. Adèle left her mother's side, marched right over to me with a big smile and reached out to shake my hand. It was great. As for her tumor, she is only a fifth of the way there, and her chances are less than 50:50 that she will survive.

Sunday, 20 February 2011

The nurse on duty called me last night for a 9 month old girl who had half swallowed an earring earlier in the day. He said he could feel it when he put his finger in her throat, but he couldn't see it or grab it. I went up. It was not in her windpipe, and she was having no trouble breathing, but she had pink-flecked foam bubbling at her lips and a fixed, startled look on her face. She was in the arms of her grandfather, who was perched on a stool. Her mother sat on a bench on the other side of the room, stifling little sobs. I pried open the child's mouth with a tongue depressor and shined a light, but I saw no foreign body. I thought—hoped—maybe they were mistaken, but when I put my finger in (in spite of her 9 months she had no teeth yet; God had this thing all thought out in advance), the tip brushed against something hard and stuck fast in the left corner at the base of her tongue, right where it curves down into the throat. We were informed that the earring had a long post. We had to keep her from swallowing it and also, in trying to get it out, keep it from slipping into the trachea. We leaned her forward and whacked her on the back good and hard. She never cried, maybe she couldn't, through any of this. That seemed to bring the metal edge forward a little, but it was still impossible to see or to grab, we could just feel it with a fingertip. Still, we were encouraged by the progress and decided that if leaning her over and whacking her did some good, then turning her upside down might do even more. So the nurse grabbed her by the heels like a newborn and I steadied her head and neck, and we whacked away. A bit more progress. We did it again. I wonder how, as she grows older, she will construe or remember this night. But at least she will grow older. We laid her belly-down on her grandfather's lap, head dangling down the side of his thigh, and I tried again. This time I was able to hook my index finger under the bottom of something and, with considerable difficulty but ultimate success, sweep it forward. Out came a metal flower—bigger than a nickel, smaller than a quarter—clanging to the floor. That's not all, I said. I swept again and a second metal flower clanged to the floor. Once more, and a half-inch pointy post clanged to the floor. And as it did, the mother's sobs across the room unstifled themselves and she cried and cried and cried and cried. I felt nothing more in the child's throat and was worried about the second post, but they assured me there had been only one. In an instant the baby fell fast asleep lying there on her grandfather's lap. This morning when I came to her on rounds she was breastfeeding happily. She stopped when I started talking to her mother and looked up at me and there was not the slightest malice in her eyes, so in spite of our torture session I think we are okay.

One of the diabetics we have followed for years, a young man now married and with a toddler, has been on Lilly insulin since he was in grade school. He works as a heavy laborer, loading and unloading trucks up on the border. A few weeks ago he got a minuscule scrape on the index finger of his right hand—he is right handed—and neglected it, something a diabetic can never let himself do. The finger swelled up and the infection festered, started creeping up his hand, then his arm. In an effort to save all of the above, and in fact his life, we had to take him to the O.R. to open the thing up, slicing right down the finger into the palm of his hand. He was put under general anesthesia for the surgery. I went over to see him when he came round afterwards. He was awake, though not quite altogether with it. He smiled brightly when I greeted him. "I have just been," he said, "to your village." "Oh?" I said. "Yes," he replied. "And it is very nice there, and the weather is beautiful, and the houses and the cars." I told him I was glad he liked it. "And my people—did you see my people?" I asked. "Oh yes," he said "and they are well. They are all very well." "That's wonderful," I said, "Thank you." He drifted off. The next morning when I went to greet him, he was sheepish, embarrassed, said he understood that he had said some things to me the day before that were nonsense, maybe bad. I assured him that he did nothing of the sort, that in fact he said nothing but the best of everything and he made me happy to hear it.

26 March 2011

The heartbreak of the week was the death of Adèle, the young retinoblastoma patient I told you about a few weeks ago, the wailer who finally came around, whose clenched fist and howl gave way to an extended hand and smile, whose smile could make my whole day. She wobbled seriously after her first two cycles of chemo, but she bounced back each time and was in good shape when we sent her over to have the cancerous eye removed. She tolerated the surgery poorly, and evidently the tumor had extended back into her brain. She had neurologic problems post-op, increased intracranial pressure with ferocious headaches, finally convulsions and death. Losing her took the wind out of me, was very hard.

Saturday, 2 July 2011

I don't know if such news reaches you, but Maiduguri, the capital of Borno State, Nigeria, our closest Nigerian city and one from which a large number of our patients come, has become a hotbed of Islamic fundamentalist terrorists—real wackos. They've been setting fires and throwing bombs indiscriminately and conducting drive-by shootings.

Sunday, 17 July 2011

Things are not looking good in Maiduguri. The Islamic fundamentalist group called Boko Haram that caused a lot of rioting, destruction and death back in 2009 has risen from the ashes and is creating havoc. Their favorite weapons appear to be IEDs and fire bombs, both aimed at any police or government authority or else just at random crowds. The main agenda of this group is to institute Sharia law nationwide (it is already in Borno State) and to get rid of every form of Western education. Children, in their view, should be taught the Quran, and that is it. (But how a child taught only the Quran will learn to build an IED they do not explain and I assume that will be problematic for them.) Hundreds have been killed. Thousands have fled, shops are shuttered, motorcycle traffic (the main means of getting around) has been forbidden. The army has been sent in, there are checkpoints everywhere. The government does not so far appear to be winning the battle. In fact as skittish soldiers shoot indiscriminately, they are making enemies of their own. All of this matters to us because Maiduguri is only 100 km from here, many of our patients come from there, a great deal of what we find in our markets comes from there, and—and—the only man we have ever found who can fix our generator reliably is from there but has now fled to Lagos. Also we are getting refugees—those seeking safety and those fleeing arrest—in our border towns, and that if it continues will be trouble.

Just before midday on a Friday in late August, a car laden with explosives barreled into the United Nations building in Nigeria's capital, Abuja. Twenty-three people were killed and over seventy others were wounded. In claiming responsibility for the attack, Boko Haram's spokesman decried police brutality and demanded the liberation of all Boko Haram prisoners.

Wednesday, 01 February 2012

Officially the borders are closed, but it appears there are enough ways around the closure for people who have a little bribe money in their pockets to get through. I have been seeing plenty of Nigerians in consultation, and they are

*occupying half our beds. Also northern Nigerians have been finding Camerou-
nian relatives and sending their families over to stay with them until the troubles
die down (when, exactly?), so we might be having a swollen population for a
while.*

*There is concern in the population and among the authorities on this side
of the border because of the bombings in Nigeria, but no panic and no real fear
that the chaos will spill over. The feeling is that the violence in Nigeria is political
and that the religious front is only a disguise used to better rally the people and
hide the real agenda from international onlookers.*

Part IV

When suffering knocks at your door and you say there is no seat for him,
he tells you not to worry because he has brought his own stool.

Chinua Achebe

BY THE END of 2012, the hospital had grown to ten hectares holding thirteen major pavilions and 120 beds that were filled as soon as they were freed. One hundred fifty outpatients were being treated every day, and up to thirty patients a day were having their cataracts surgically removed and replaced with lens implants. The hospital's laboratory was the best equipped in the Far North. A 65 kVA Caterpillar generator provided back-up electrical power, and water cisterns and overhead tanks held a reserve of nearly 200,000 liters of water. The hospital retained the allure of a rural no-frills facility, but from Cameroon and around the world it attracted nursing students, medical students, and specialty residents hoping to receive training in its unique setting. A panoply of diseases including measles, polio, meningococcal meningitis, neonatal tetanus, leprosy, Guinea worm, and trachoma had disappeared from our district; the only patients we still saw with these conditions came from other countries, where communities stretched beyond the reach of our preventive services.

More children than ever—and more girls than ever—were enrolled in school, and there were now fifty-one primary schools for them to attend. The Women's Center hosted classes daily and had a chicken farm to generate its own income. Several secondary schools, including one for technical training, had been built. Cell phones were ubiquitous. Motorcycles were taking the place of bicycles.

Hopeful and focused on moving ever forward, we were dismissive of the whirlwind building up across the border and had no idea it was about to blow our way.

I Wonder Who Will Deliver *Her* First Child

Wednesday, 09, January 2013

Friday [we received] a 70 year old man who had fallen out of a tree. What, you may ask, and we did, was a 70 year old man doing climbing a tree? He was picking fruit, the family said, and maybe he was. But more likely he wasn't. More likely he was attacked, or hit by a motorcycle, and he and the family, not wanting to get tangled up with the law, decided to call it a fall from a tree. Not a scratch on him, but his sternum is depressed into the middle of his chest cavity and his spinal cord is crushed at the same level, so he has no sensation and is paralyzed from the chest down, and this, for whatever time he has left, will not change. There is little we can do for him. These kinds of cases are particularly heart wrenching because in the initial hours or sometimes days the patient in spite of his pain is almost euphoric (I survived!) and while we want to share his euphoria, if only to encourage him, we know too well what is going gradually to dawn on him, that life as he knew it is over and only agony of the most excruciating sort lies ahead.

On a Wednesday morning in mid-January we were surprised by a visit from three young American men. Somehow managing to look both spit-and-polish neat and scruffy at the same time—their beards, perhaps, accounted for the scruffiness—they introduced themselves to us as United States Navy officers who had been stationed in Maroua since October. There was nothing in their dress that indicated they were military. They wore no insignia and appeared to be bearing no arms. They claimed they were training Cameroonian rapid intervention teams, and they had been asked by the United States ambassador to come to Kolofata to collect information about us and the hospital. They took photographs and asked many questions, answering our own in the vaguest possible way. They reminded me of my own brothers at that age: fit and strong, pleased with their strength, wide-eyed and innocent, ready to take on the world. Before leaving they gave us their phone numbers and e-mail addresses and encouraged us to contact them if we ever needed the slightest thing or had any doubt about our safety. Not knowing what they might be getting at, I was nevertheless happy with this and unexpectedly heartened to learn that American military men were only a hundred kilometers away. But I wondered why, really, they were here and what they might know but did not care to say.

Monday, 28 January 2013

One of [our recent] newborns [is] the baby of a woman we delivered 18 years ago. She came to the maternity ward with that carnet she was issued when she was a day old and receiving her first vaccination. It takes my breath away when I see these kinds of things. All those years, all that life lived, all the trauma and the joy and the heartbreak and the milestones packed in, and it went by in a flash. And this baby born Thursday night—who will be here to deliver her first child?

Saturday, 2 Feb. We are doing our month-end reports and I discovered yesterday evening that in January we set an all-time record for number of patients seen in consultation in one month. This delights me—not that we set a record but that it didn't feel like we were setting a record.

Friday, 08 February 2013

I had a visit from a judge yesterday. (Oh no, thought Myra, reflecting on the dozens of things we have been accused of, they have finally found a hanging rope.) I did not know he was a judge, only that he and a woman had come from Mora to see me about a case. I was in the middle of three simultaneous emergencies—a badly burned child, a difficult delivery and an ultrasound Marion [our French medical resident] was doing and having a hard time interpreting—in three different corners of the hospital—but I got them all wrapped up or looked after as quickly as I could and went up to receive our visitors.

He introduced himself as a judge and gave me his name and then indicated the (nameless) thin meek woman beside him as the prosecutor from Mora. She did not look like she could prosecute a fly, so I don't know if she was the real prosecutor or a clerk sent to fill in. I asked how I might help them.

"Two people, a man and a woman, have been receiving AIDS treatment in your hospital for some years," he said. "They are not married, but they were a couple, and the father of the young woman has sued the man for having infected his daughter with the virus. We would like to know if you can tell us if this is true."

Of course I could not, as he must have known.

"Well then, we would like you to tell us which one started receiving treatment first."

His upper lip had a tremor, and I wondered if this was a defect, a nervous tic, or a sign of suppressed anger.

I told him that was privileged information and it was out of the question for me to divulge.

The lip twitch increased in amplitude as he bounced in his chair and cranked up the volume: Did I not know who he was? Did I not know what power he possessed? Who was I to impede justice? Was I covering for this man? He could force me to do anything he wanted, did I not know that? etc. I told him his tirade was inappropriate and asked him to calm down—which only got him going at twice the volume and double the twitch. He had the power to confiscate every document in this hospital if he wanted! He was a judge! After fifteen minutes of this he abruptly slammed shut his file, rose, and stormed out of my office—not a handshake, not a thank-you, not a good-bye: in this culture a grievous omission.

So next time we will check him at the gate for that hanging rope, for surely next time he will not leave it behind.

Tuesday, 12 Feb. Yesterday was the dreaded Youth Day and so we dutifully spent several hours sitting on hard plastic chairs squinting into the sun watching thousands of schoolchildren march past, our eardrums ringing from, on the right, groups of traditional drummers drumming; on the left an MC babbling nonstop into a microphone; in the front, children singing at the top of their lungs as they marched past; and overhead piped godawful rock music. By the time it was all over I felt not unlike I feel after a 44 hour trans-Mediterranean/ transatlantic flight.

Sunday, 17 February 2013

Letter number 500. That is a lot of ink, a lot of pages—though not nearly as many as you have written, Mom, and sent the other way.

The War Is Going to Come to Cameroon

ON TUESDAY, FEBRUARY 19, I was finishing an ultrasound exam on a pregnant woman when Marion, our French medical resident, came into the ultrasound room. She was staring at her phone.

"A French family," she said, "has been kidnapped from Dabanga and taken to Nigeria." Dabanga was just north, not far from Kolofata. Marion was agitated; her father and sister had arrived the day before from France for a visit. We made phone calls to as many sources as we could think of, but all we could discover was that earlier that day armed men on motorcycles had pounced as the family left the game park lodge in Waza, where they had spent the night. Four children ranging from four to twelve years old, the mother, the father, and the father's brother had been taken.

In that instant I knew that just as life for that kidnapped family had pivoted, everything for us, for Kolofata, and for the hospital had changed as well. Despite reassurances from Boko Haram that they had no interest in anything outside Nigeria's borders, the war was going to come to Cameroon.

The French Embassy in Yaoundé ordered any French citizen who was within thirty kilometers of the Nigerian border to leave the country or come farther inside. Kolofata was eleven kilometers from the border, and in addition to Marion and her family, we were hosting four French men and women engaged in different activities at the hospital. Before the day was over, two militarized Land Cruisers and a squad of heavily armed Cameroon Rapid Intervention Brigade troops, or BIR, had arrived in Kolofata. Their assignment was to guard any foreigners still in Kolofata and to take out any who were willing to leave.

Over the next several days, all of them left except Myra and me.

If ransom demands for the kidnapped family were made, they were not announced to the public. Days and then weeks started passing, and the crisis dragged on, and one by one our expected visitors from Europe and North America canceled their plans: nursing and medical students, medical residents, a radiologist/ultrasonographer, other doctors, an information technologist, a researcher.

Thursday, 28 February 2013

The hostages as I write remain unreleased. I assume the French/Nigerian/ Cameroonian governments know where they are and are biding their time, but maybe not. Security on this side of the border has been beefed up. When we were in Maroua last week we saw armed and helmeted military men in unfamiliar places, particularly at the corners going into and out of the city. Armed patrols— some men conspicuous in army or gendarme uniform, others in disguise—keep an eye on Kolofata, and the two of us have our own little band of bodyguards, strapping young soldiers with rifles slung from their shoulders.

My faith in these latter was shaken by two incidents. We in particular and the population in general have been warned to be wary of strangers, [especially] unfamiliar men on motorcycles, lurking about. At mid-morning on Tuesday, the man who guards our main gate at the hospital came to tell me that a strange fellow on a motorcycle had been coming to the hospital every day for the last week or so, just hanging out at the gate. He was neither a patient nor a caregiver, he wasn't a taxi man and he wasn't a food seller. He was not from around here, no one knew him, and he seemed to have no purpose being here. The area just outside the hospital gate is an easy place for lurking and for information gathering. Over the years a small market has sprung up there to cater to our large clientele, it is where motorcycles and cars park when they bring patients, and staff and patients' families go there to eat. I suggested to our army guys that they check him out, and they did. Apparently he did not cooperate with their questioning, would not produce any ID, would not tell them where he was from, and so they escorted him to the local gendarme station. I gather the local gendarmes got no further with him, for the next morning the Commandant called me to tell me he was taking him to Mora.

So that was okay as far as it went—I just hope we are not bringing all this grief to an innocent man—but the more worrying incident happened at the end of the day. Our "workday" goes from 7:30 to 3:30, and most days we do manage to wrap up more or less on time. The four night nurses come on and the ten day nurses leave. One night guard comes at 3:30, the other not until 6. The pharmacists, promoters and all other auxiliary staff leave. I usually stay for another couple hours to do my evening visit of inpatients and, if things are calm, to attack paperwork.

Tuesday was a heavy day and we had to keep our heads down and scramble all day to get patients in and out. No one got out on time, but by 4:00 people started to leave, and by 4:15 when I went out to have a last word with one of our pharmacists I discovered that all the staff had gone. The night nurses were off in different wards. The night guard was near the front of the compound taking down the flag. Two of our soldiers were sitting on a bench on the front verandah of the OPD. My office is in the back of the OPD.

I went in there and started sorting through a pile of papers on my desk and I had not even sat down when a wiry little man—could have been a clone of Ahmadinejad, except with grayer, disheveled hair—burst into my office through the front door. People here would call him white, but he was swarthy, middle-Eastern, with a mustache and a beard and a constant smile that pulled the sides of his mouth out rather than up, in a straight line rather than a curve. He was brandishing an ID card, a Cameroonian ID card. He held this out to me and I took it, but I was so astonished by his bursting in on me like that (where were my soldiers??) that I barely looked at it. I thought later that that probably made no difference, for if he was up to no good, the card was surely a fake anyway, but at the time, as the minutes passed, I was cursing myself for not having looked better at the card. Anyway, he had a running monologue: he was from Lebanon, he had been "in education" in Yaoundé for years, he was now up here looking to open a restaurant, Middle Eastern food, but he wasn't sure Africans would like Middle Eastern food, but he would do it without too much—what do you call it—fat, and he had heard so much about this hospital, a big hospital, "mostly" Nigerian patients, lots of foreigners working here, and he was thinking of opening a restaurant in Maroua, but he thought after all why not here. All of this said with that knifeblade smile. I broke in from time to time, said he seemed thirsty and regretted I had no cold water to offer him. Yes, he said, he was, but that was understandable since he had just come a long distance on a motorcycle. He had left the front door of my office open and for this I was grateful, but every once in a while a breeze would catch it and swing it nearly closed and I kept wondering what I would do if it snapped shut. I also kept wondering where the soldiers were and how this guy knew exactly where to come to find me and why he waited until all the staff and patients had gone before he did and what, really, he was doing here.

I did not feel threatened, only puzzled and maybe worried that I was not smart enough to figure this out. As luck would have it, at that moment, John, our gardener/part-time driver/generator keeper, came in through my back door to hand in the generator key. I had told him fifteen minutes before all this to go home, and I had thought him gone, but he had not yet done something that needed doing on the generator, hence his return to hand in the key. Confusion froze his face when he walked in and saw me standing there with Ahmadinejad, but I told him to come in, have a seat, I would get to him in a minute, and he hesitated at first but then got my point and came in and had a seat. Whether coincidence or not, this seemed to mark the end of my visitor's visit, and he said he would be moving on. And out he went, and I told John to go and ever so delicately tell one of the soldiers that they might want to keep an eye on him. But apparently they did not. John did, however, as the man wandered around the compound a while, found a plastic kettle with which to do his ablutions, prayed behind the male ward (though it was not prayer time) and finally left. Someone the next morning told me he took the motorcycle down our hill, got stuck in the sand, and finally hitched a ride (or were they waiting for him?) with a big lorry on the main road loaded with pipes and other hardware.

So. Was he an innocent entrepreneur surveying the marketplace, hoping to open a restaurant? Was he sent by some extremist group to scout plausible targets, be they places or people? Was his odd comment that he did not think he would be opening his restaurant here meant to reassure me? Was the whole visit meant, rather, to scare me? Who knows. The next day the Commandant of the local Gendarmes called me to express his fury that I had not called him immediately. He had a point and humbly I had to admit that, but I also told him that I thought telling the soldiers, who after all were armed and had the guy right there in front of them, was enough and they would do whatever needed to be done or inform whomever needed to be informed. The Commandant only sighed and growled.

Sunday, 3 March. AA came on Friday night, and we had a nice dinner with him, Kolofata's main chief, and a few of our local elites last night. The food and drink were good, but the conversation turned the whole evening around issues of security and insecurity, the disintegration of Nigeria, the tragedy of all this spilling into Cameroun and what must be done to stop it. I'm afraid none of us left the table feeling very reassured.

Northeastern Nigeria's Borno State, the state that borders most of our district, is the modern-day administrative remnant of what was once the powerful empire of Kanem-Bornu. Home of the Kanuri tribe, the Kanem-Bornu Empire was established around 1380 and reached its apogee in the late sixteenth century under Idris Alooma, a warrior-statesman and devout Muslim intent on extending the influence of Islam throughout his empire and beyond. Kanuris tended trade routes leading from sub-Saharan Africa to North Africa and Mecca. Ostrich feathers, salt, animal hides, cotton, and kola nuts were among the goods traded out of Africa, but the most valuable and profitable were slaves. To ensure a constant supply of slaves, Kanuri raiders mounted on armored horses and armed with machetes and spears invaded villages, looted homes, stole livestock, abducted people, and burned whatever was left in their wake. With each conquest their kingdom grew until it englobed most of the central African Sahel.

Following the death of Idris in 1603 the Kanem-Bornu Empire entered a period of slow decline. Successive famines and conquests by other tribes led to the disintegration of the kingdom. By the nineteenth century, Kanuri power had devolved to lesser chiefs with fiefdoms scattered throughout what would become northeastern Nigeria, northern Cameroon, and parts of Niger and Chad.

The descendants of the old Kanem-Bornu Empire remained refractory to the same development sought so avidly by people of neighboring cultures. With rare exceptions they disdained formal education for their children, and they tolerated first colonial and then national government without supporting it or engaging with it.

Mostly, they wanted to be left alone. They wanted to hoe their fields and look after their sheep and goats, and they wanted their children to follow in their footsteps. Parents came to realize that a child whose formal education taught him to speak French or English and to read and write and calculate was unlikely to be content remaining in the village looking after goats or hoeing half-acre fields. The more ardent among them reasoned that since the Quran and the Hadith explained everything anyone needed to know in order to live a perfect life in a perfect society, education not founded on these ancient sacred sources was not only unnecessary but harmful. They felt that so-called Western education, with its emphasis on unbridled exposure to knowledge and on the development of critical thinking, went far beyond basic Islamist precepts and should therefore be forbidden.

Into this fertile ground were planted seeds of political discontent, as different factions within Nigerian politics vied for power. The less scrupulous among them saw no reason not to exploit the North's Islamist extremists, and so they harnessed the fundamentalists' manpower and energy to their own runaway wagons in the hope of wreaking enough havoc to destabilize Nigeria's existing southern-dominated power structure.

Soon after the dawn of the twenty-first century, these various forces within northern Nigerian society began to coalesce around a number of political and religious leaders. One of them, Muhammed Yusuf, was a compelling Muslim preacher whose sermons and teachings decried Western education. Parents mistrustful of government schools were happy to send their children to Yusuf's madrassa to be instructed instead in his fundamentalist interpretation of the Quran and extreme libertarian view of government. In time his followers reached a critical mass.

Absurdly, what sparked the conversion of a radical but basically pacific group of people into a raging mob and then over the years into a well-armed, disciplined, vicious militia was the passing of a law requiring motorcyclists to wear helmets. The fundamentalists were against this law and refused to comply. Nigerian law enforcement officers, not known for their high regard for human rights, reacted to their refusal with a heavy hand, and one thing led to another: demonstrations, riots, killings, burnings. Eventually Muhammed Yusuf, the Muslim preacher, was arrested and, stripped and bound, summarily executed by his law enforcement captors. This was in 2009.

Far from silencing the extremists, and with no shortage of men ready to take his place, the extrajudicial killing of Yusuf sounded a piercing battle cry that crescendoed rapidly. In rampages reminiscent of the old Kanem-Bornu Empire, bands of men—on motorcycle now rather than horseback and wielding Kalashnikovs and grenades rather than machetes and spears—began raiding villages, looting homes, stealing livestock, abducting and assassinating people, and burning whatever was left in their wake.

The objectives of the sect appeared to be threefold: first, to defend themselves and their faith (as they saw it) by killing members of the armed forces, Christians, and anyone, including other Muslims, whom they considered traitors to their cause; second, to liberate by whatever means necessary any of their members who had been imprisoned; and third, to destabilize the region by fomenting maximum terror and disorder.

In many ways, Kolofatans were historically oriented more westward toward Nigeria than eastward toward the interior of their own country. In addition to the proclivity of Kanuris to look to Maiduguri, the capital of Borno State, as their own capital, goods in Kolofata were bought and sold with Nigerian currency. The district's two main markets were both on the other side of the border. Kolofatan youth with a sense of wanderlust aspired to seek work in Lagos, Nigeria's former capital, rather than in Cameroon's big cities. Kolofatan parents commonly sought Nigerian husbands for their daughters.

It was also impossible to separate perpetrators evading capture from true refugees fleeing persecution. Cameroonian villagers knew who among them were foreigners, but since in most cases they were members of their own extended families, newcomers were concealed from the authorities no matter which way suspicions pointed. At first this protection was offered, however reluctantly, out of a sense of family loyalty. Later, as it dawned on Cameroonians that their own peace and survival might be at stake, it was offered out of terror of reprisal should protection be withdrawn.

Youth in both Nigeria and Cameroon were co-opted to the extremists' cause. Wooed by promises of recruiting fees, guns, and glory, uneducated teenaged boys whose tame predictable futures were locked into village life were seduced with alarming ease. Most had little knowledge of Islam and were motivated less by religion or ideology than by the prospect of money and power.

Violence spilled, like a toxic brew bubbling in a cauldron too small to contain it, over the border into northern Cameroon. During the final months of 2012 we started to see more and more battered pickup trucks with Nigerian license plates rumble into town. They were packed with people and their belongings—pots, blankets, bundles of cloth, straw mats and thin foam mattresses, axes and hoes, burlap sacks of grain. Sometimes we saw groups of people on foot: women mostly, trekking toward uncertain destinations, babies wrapped on their backs, toddlers trailing at their sides, loads piled improbably high on their heads.

Traveling from one village to another within our part of Cameroon became difficult and fraught with danger. Routes used by arms smugglers cut through our district. Military checkpoints sprang up, manned by soldiers and police trained to be suspicious of everyone. Dusk-to-dawn curfews were instated throughout.

Suspected sympathizers of terrorists were arrested by law enforcement officers; suspected informants were hunted down and killed by the other side.

Saturday, 9th of March, 2013

We are being followed everywhere by armed soldiers. As far as I know, there have been no further incidents since the kidnapping a few weeks ago, but also no word on the whereabouts or fate of the hostages. Peace Corps has closed all of their posts up here and a lot of missionaries and others of various nationalities have left.

We had a horrific case come in late Thursday. A young woman of about twenty-five, an epileptic, fell into a fire face first. Actually, the initial story was that she fell into a fire. She sustained skull-deep burns over her entire face and deep burns over the front of her neck. Her eyelids melted together, her nostrils melted shut. Her lips are so swollen they have retracted from her teeth. Her swollen tongue fills most of her mouth. Her entire face is charcoal black and just as hard. Assuming she stays alive, it will take several days for that charred crust to start peeling away from the skull, and God only knows what will happen then.

She cannot have fallen into a fire, because flames lick and burns are not so localized and well delineated. She had not even first degree burns on the back of her head or neck, nor on her hands or anywhere else on her body. When I pointed out to the family how odd this seemed, the story changed: she did not fall into a fire but rather into a pot of boiling water. Face down into a pot of boiling water. No, no one was at home at the time. Her father-in-law found her. I'm still not sure this is plausible. How is it she was in boiling water for long enough to burn her whole face down to the skull and yet show no signs of near drowning? I have no idea what happened to her but I don't think it is what the family is saying.

It is not even mid-March and already we have been having water problems on and off and electrical outages pretty much every day. It is going to be a long hot hot season and a long dark rainy season. One of the problems most annoying is that when the electricity goes out and eventually comes back on it goes out and comes back on with a bang, doing damage to equipment.

Another of our concerns at the moment is that the French company that makes our anti-snake venom has once again stopped production. If we can't figure something out people are going to die.

Do They Want to Kill You or Abduct You?

On March 12, a French cable news television station, France 24, reported that seven foreigners kidnapped by Islamist extremists from Bauchi State—this kidnapping had been three days before the French family was taken from

Cameroon—had been killed by their captors. This was shocking news. Bauchi is in Nigeria, but not far from us, and many of our patients were from there.

The following evening, Wednesday, March 13, I came down from the hospital just before six o'clock and was surprised to find that in addition to the old group there was a new group of soldiers at the house. I wondered why there were so many.

We had just finished our chicken-and-potatoes dinner when my phone rang. The screen showed an unknown Orange cell phone number. I answered, *"Allô?"* and was surprised when the voice transmitted from the other end was American-accented English.

"Is this Dr. Ellen Einterz?"

I asked who was calling.

"This is Scott Irwin of the American Embassy in Yaoundé. Is this Dr. Ellen Einterz?" he asked again.

"It is."

He spoke slowly, clearly. "I am calling to inform you that the embassy has received information from a credible source that a group is planning to kidnap you and your Canadian colleague. Soon. Probably very soon."

I stood up with deliberate calm and went over to the desk to find a pen and paper. "Scott Irwin," I wrote. "US Embassy. Kidnap."

Scott Irwin went on. "Right now I want to get some numbers from you, I want to give you some numbers, and I want to know if you would agree to have us send a team in to get you out. They are ready to come now. Are you at home?"

I told him I was.

"I want you to stay there, don't go anywhere, don't go out. I understand that you have some military personnel with you. Is that right? Are they armed?"

"We used to have four," I told him, "but this afternoon they seem to have multiplied, maybe ten. Yes, they are armed, or they have rifles at least."

He asked if there was another telephone number at which he could reach me in case this one did not go through. I gave him Myra's.

"Can we send a team to get you?" he asked once more.

"No, I don't think so," I answered, trying not to sound ungrateful. "I don't suppose you can tell me what it was you were told or how you got the information?"

"I'm sorry, ma'am; no, I can't, but it is from a reliable source we have used in the past. We consider it a credible threat, and we are taking it very seriously."

This seemed to me so improbable; I had to ask, "But it could be a hoax, couldn't it, or someone wanting to cause trouble?"

"Yes, it could, but we are taking it seriously, and we advise you to take it seriously." He was pleasant, but unyielding. He gave me the embassy number and extension and said that the security officer from the embassy would be calling me shortly. Then the phone went dead.

Throughout this call Myra had been looking at me in an anxious sort of way. After my phone went dead I relayed to her our conversation.

"Oh," she said.

We took the dishes into the kitchen, which was across our small sandy courtyard—I couldn't help noticing how dark it was outside—and started washing them. Soon the phone rang again.

I answered, and the man on the other end identified himself as the security officer for the American Embassy in Yaoundé, and he confirmed who I was. He repeated the information: credible threat; kidnapping; you and your Canadian colleague; we have a team ready to get you out; would you be willing to leave until the threat has passed?

For the threat to pass, I suggested, could take forever.

He had no answer to this. He asked about the soldiers around us: were they armed, how many were there, were they ordinary military or were they BIR. He repeated, "This threat is credible and we are taking it very seriously. You are a private citizen and as such I cannot order you to do anything, but let me just tell you that if you were an employee of the United States government, I would order you to leave right now."

I thanked him and told him I understood; I then explained that we had a pretty big hospital and a busy health service, and I was the only doctor for a large population, and I really did not think it was a good idea to leave.

"You know we have pulled all Peace Corps volunteers out of the areas bordering Nigeria?" he asked.

I told him I had heard. I did not add that I knew the volunteers had been instructed to pack up quietly, quickly, and leave. Tell no one, they had been ordered, say no good-byes, just leave.

He asked, "Do you have a sponsoring agency?"

I told him about VICS and wondered aloud if Amadou Ali was aware of this.

"If Monsieur Ali doesn't already know, I will be informing him immediately."

I told him that we had not heard from the Canadian High Commission, which seemed strange. Did they know? Why had Myra not been contacted?

"We ourselves have just learned," he replied, "and the Canadians might not know yet. I will call my counterpart at the Canadian High Commission as soon as we hang up, and I am sure they will be contacting her this evening."

"Am I to tell the soldiers guarding us what you have told me?"

At first he said no; then he said their commanders must already know, since they had reinforced their team. So I should go ahead and tell the guards that we had been contacted by the American embassy and been advised to advise them to be vigilant.

"Can I call Amadou Ali?"

"Yes, by all means."

Then he said he was sorry, but there was someone at the door and he had to hang up. He assured me he would be calling again.

About fifteen minutes later a man identifying himself as Dan Giroux called on Myra's phone. She put it on speaker. He was from the Canadian High Commission in Yaoundé, he said, and he went through the same message with her. He said the high commission was going on what the Americans told them. They were taking the threat seriously, and if she wanted to leave, the American team would come get her out even if the American doctor did not wish to go.

Myra mentioned the doubling of the guard as of today and said that we seemed to be quite well protected. I scribbled a note on a napkin and passed it to Myra, telling her to ask if the threat was a general one against a place or a group of people or if it was a specific threat against the two of us. She asked this, and Dan said he did not know but would try to find out.

After offering some words of encouragement and instructions to call if she felt the slightest need, he hung up. Shortly after, he called again to relay to her the information they had received, that the threat was specific regarding the two of us. He added that the people making the threat were aware that we were being guarded by armed military.

Myra asked how they thought they could kidnap us if we were being guarded.

"Easy," he said. "You have ten men around you. The kidnappers come with thirty."

We hung up, and half an hour later my phone rang again. This time it was a woman with a southern American accent. She identified herself as Erica Lewis and explained to me that the United States Embassy's raison d'être is to ensure the safety of American citizens in the country and that her job at that moment was to convince me to leave Kolofata. "We will take you and your Canadian colleague to Maroua—we are ready to come get you right now—and you probably would only have to stay there for a few days, just until the threat passes."

I asked her how she knew the threat would pass in a few days.

Pause. "Well, I don't," she replied.

She said she was a mother, and she would not want her daughter staying put in a situation like this. I guessed she was twenty or thirty years younger than me, but I understood what she was trying to say.

"We know you are dedicated and all that. But just for a few days," she added.

When I told her, as we had told the others, that we were already being guarded round the clock by armed military personnel and that the guard had just been increased, she reminded me that that was no guarantee of anything; people who had been protected by larger guards than ours had been kidnapped, or worse.

I wondered what her job title was. "Anyway," I said, "it is night now and not very wise to be going anywhere. Would it be OK if I talk it over with Myra and we come to a decision by tomorrow?"

She said she would call me first thing in the morning.

I called Amadou Ali, told him everything, expressed my reluctance to leave, and asked him if he had any idea where this was coming from.

He did and he had been aware of the threats against us and against Kolofata in general since the day before. "The Americans and the French *et les autres* do not understand everything, and they have to do what they feel they have to do. These *terroristes* know that they only have to make threats. People get scared, they leave."

He seemed to be echoing my thoughts and then added, "Don't get me wrong. We feel this is serious, and we are taking extraordinary steps to be sure you will be safe if you decide to stay. But if you are uneasy and want to leave, my house in Maroua is open to you. You can stay there for however long you want."

I told him I did not want to go anywhere. I wanted to stay in Kolofata.

"*C'est ça,*" he answered, his tone implying that it was the only logical conclusion. "Then we will see to it that you are protected." As if in an afterthought he asked, "Do they want to kill you or abduct you?"

This gave me a jolt. "Abduct, I'm told."

"Well then, OK. The men protecting you—they can do that, they will not let that happen. But be careful, keep your eyes open. Anyone can pretend to be a patient, and it is not impossible that someone among your own staff could be involved in something."

I assured him I was aware of this.

He told me he had to leave the country that night for a few days, but he would be back Saturday. He gave me the names of people I should contact for any questions or problems in the meantime, and he told me that even in Europe his usual phone numbers would work, I could call him any time.

Fifteen minutes later Myra's phone rang. A man speaking French identified himself as Capitaine Paul. She asked him how he got her phone number, and he said he got it from the embassy. It became evident he thought he was talking to me. Myra did not correct him. He told her that four BIRs would be arriving shortly on motorcycles and would be charged with ensuring our personal safety at all times. They were to be at our side everywhere we went. He said that he would be calling the commander of the squad outside to inform him of this.

I was suspicious. What if these four were in fact our kidnappers, disguised as personal bodyguards, coming on motorcycles to "ensure our personal safety" by taking us away? It would be a clever idea. I got the number from Myra's received-calls log and phoned him back. I asked for more information and for the name of his superior, and something convinced me that he was genuine. I thanked him and relaxed. I then called the commandant of the Kolofata gendarmerie to make sure he was in the loop. He was and had been since earlier that afternoon. I realized we were the last to be informed of the threat against us.

About forty minutes later Capitaine Paul called back to say five BIRs—he had added a fifth—had arrived in our compound.

We began to look around our small house and wonder what we would take if we had to leave suddenly, either as kidnap victims or as travelers being escorted to Maroua for an indefinite but at least more comfortable stay. If we were kidnapped, would our abductors let us take something with us? If we asked, would they say yes, just so they could then relieve us of whatever we considered most valuable?

I had an overnight satchel whose contents I never unpacked, and to these I added two dresses, a pad of paper, a few paperbacks, and a book of poetry. To her bag, Myra added malaria pills and half a dozen tubes of lip balm. We charged our phones and laptops.

I wondered how they would do it. Would they ambush us in our car, the way they did the French family? Would they send a fake emergency to the hospital in the middle of the night? Would they break down our door at two in the morning? Come through the ceiling? Smash the window? Would they burst in with guns blazing, or would they be stealthy and smooth and secrete us away?

We uncapped a can of household insecticide and put it on the table beside the door: the best we could do in the way of a weapon. Aim for the eyes, I told Myra. She also put a stout stick and an iron bar by the door. I wasn't sure I could wield either one to any meaningful effect, but they were there. I set an easy-to-get-into dress beside my bed. We put temporary drapes over some of our less protected windows, made sure the doors were locked and the outside lights on.

Finally we called it a night. I slept fitfully, hearing the fall of every leaf. Each time I woke up I mulled over choices, and by morning the two of us had decided we had no option but to stay. We figured that if we really were the targets of a kidnapping, the kidnappers would get to us no matter where we were. They would follow us to Maroua if need be, and in Maroua we probably would not have the heavy guard we had in Kolofata. On the other hand, if all they really cared about was to scare us and chase us away, showing their power by damaging the hospital or Kolofata or the thousands of people who depended on us, then by fleeing we would achieve their objective for them. Leaving, it seemed to us, had nothing to recommend it.

I was happy to see the dawn. We went through our usual routine. I watched the news—the world had a new pope—and after eating breakfast we headed to the hospital. At seven thirty, just as I was beginning morning rounds, Erica Lewis called, greeted, and asked if we had made a decision. I told her that five more BIRs had arrived in the night. We felt we were in good hands and had decided to stay. I got the impression while talking to her that the embassy was satisfied that, should anything happen to us, there was now documented proof that the government had tried to get us out. I also realized that having declined its help, we would henceforth be on our own. A little later the Canadian High Commission called and held a similar conversation with Myra.

Friday, 15 March 2013

I read two of your letters and let me tell you again how much I love them. When I pick up a letter of yours and sit back to read it, I feel the preciousness of the time you took to write it, and I hear your voice talking just to me, and it is like you are right here beside me, and I love that. As I read I know that your own hand touched the very page I am touching, so it is almost like a little piece of you folded itself into that envelope (another reason I hate it when they open my mail) and made its way all the way here.

Our compound has turned into a military camp as the original four or five soldiers we had guarding us have become nineteen. I do not know what their exact orders are, but they are all armed and keep watch round the clock and accompany us at all times wherever we go. Not all of them at once, but enough. They can be stealthy and mysterious in the way they appear all of a sudden. Our hospital sits on a 10-acre compound and we have thirteen main pavilions, all with doors along the front and the back, and I go in and out of them in unpredictable order depending on what is happening. They don't follow me into the wards but stand a respectful twenty or so yards back. With all our trees, I don't always see them unless I look. What I find amazing is that I can go into one end of a ward, meander through the rooms and come out the other end on the other side and there is always a camouflage-clad, rifle-toting soldier standing there, a respectful distance back, as if he knew exactly where I was going to come out.

In the current state of things it is particularly disconcerting on a dark night to have the lights suddenly go out, and my first, ridiculous thought is always, Okay, this is it. Who cut the cable!

Water problems are getting steadily worse.

On March 18, France 24 reported having received the audio portion of a video released by the captors of the French hostages. They were demanding release of all Boko Haram prisoners in Nigeria and Cameroon. The father of the kidnapped family spoke briefly, declaring that his family was faring poorly. Living conditions, he said, were harsh, they were sick, and he did not think they would be able to hold out much longer. The captors insisted that they were capable of striking anywhere in Cameroon if they liked, they were prepared to kidnap more foreigners, and they were ready to start sending suicide bombers as well if their demands were not met.

The chief of Kolofata came to see me at the hospital one afternoon, and we chatted about the anarchy in Nigeria, the likelihood of lawlessness spilling over even more into Cameroon. In northern Nigeria many traditional chiefs had been killed by outlaws seeking to strike any symbol of authority. He told me he could easily become a target too. "But I am just a person," he said. "You," he nodded toward me, "you are merchandise."

Amadou Ali was calling every two or three days to see if everything was OK. "You are still in Kolofata?" he would ask every time, and I would wonder if he half expected me to say no.

Monday 25 March 2013

The woman I wrote to you about a few weeks ago, the epileptic who burned off her entire face, is still alive. Her whole forehead is nothing but skull. Her nose is gone, her upper lip too, and half or three quarters of her lower lip. Her cheeks and chin—the flesh on them—are gone, though there is a thin muscle layer that looks like it will survive if she does. Her eyes have been burned blind and she has no eyelids but the globes are still there and also might survive in some form. She is stoic beyond all belief. She can't eat because she can't chew or close her mouth and also because the remaining bit of lip (it is not actually the lip, just a chunk of flesh whose surface has disappeared) is still so raw, but she can drink, she talks, she walks around if someone guides her.

One patient we have been really happy with is a baby girl born prematurely in one of our health centers a little over a month ago and brought to us weighing all of 800 grams—that is a good deal less than 2 pounds. I can't remember ever having an 800 gram preemie survive in our hospital so I'm pretty sure this would be a first.

Thursday, 11 April 2013

We have a young man on bed suffering from multiple shotgun wounds to the back of his legs and buttocks. He was sleeping in his home with his four year old son beside him when gunmen burst into his room and raked them both. The boy died on the spot. The father survived, and will survive, but he was a wreck—psychologically—when he arrived. He is from Nigeria. There is a lot of vengeance killing going on in Nigeria. For one thing the extremists have a mob mentality—if you are not for us you are against us—and for another petty and not so petty criminals are using the "holy war" to camouflage their criminal activity and to settle scores.

Who Knows What They Are Eating

ON APRIL 19, two months to the day after the kidnapping, a spokesman for the office of the president in Yaoundé announced to the press that the French family had been released, unharmed, and had arrived in Yaoundé. There were short glimpses of the family on television. Only the French channels were carrying the story, in bright red breaking-news headlines, because the American and English channels were preoccupied with the manhunt that followed the bombings at the

Boston marathon. In Yaoundé, the two men, the father and his brother, wore the same shirts they had been wearing the day they were kidnapped. Their hair and beards were long and scraggly and made them look like twins. Their pants hung from cinched belts. The mother's eyes were sunken in darkened orbits, and the tendons in her neck were taut and vulnerable. But they were all alive, and they were free.

The violence in Nigeria escalated after the release of the hostages. In Baga 143 people were reported killed in a rampage, scores more in Maiduguri and Bama. In Banki, police and other government office buildings were burned to the ground. Militants began commandeering private vehicles at will. The chief of Duptchari and his brother, cousins of Amadou Ali, were gunned down for refusing to hand over a vehicle that did not even belong to them. Dusk-to-dawn curfews were enforced. Families fleeing the violence and uncertainty found refuge wherever they could, usually with distant relatives in one of our villages, sometimes in makeshift shacks, sometimes in the riverbed. The hospital received victims of burns and gunshot wounds, many of them children.

Unverifiable rumors started that a substantial ransom—2.5 million dollars? 3.5 million dollars? 7 million dollars?—and the freeing of an undisclosed number of prisoners from Cameroonian jails had preceded the release of the French family from captivity. This news was not cheering. Even 2.5 million dollars would recruit a lot of guerilla fighters and buy a lot of weapons.

In mid-May Goodluck Jonathan, the president of Nigeria, declared a state of emergency in three northeastern states, including the state bordering Kolofata. Elected governors were sidelined and replaced by army officers. In several neighborhoods twenty-four-hour curfews were imposed. Helicopters, fighter jets, and tanks were sent in. The bombing of terrorist training camps began. For some people this action fueled hope that the government of Nigeria was finally going to take matters in hand. For others it signaled another step toward the outbreak of civil—and possibly regional—war.

American military were in Maroua training Cameroonian special forces. French military were in Chad and also in northern Cameroon. The diplomatic community in Yaoundé and beyond was convinced that Cameroon was nowhere near up to the task of protecting its borders and that it would be years before the North lost the label of a no-go zone for foreigners.

In a meeting in Maroua with US envoys, Myra and I were given forms to fill out so that in the event we were kidnapped and held for ransom the embassy would be able to ascertain if we were alive. We had to write down, among other things, five proof-of-life facts that only we and our closest relatives would know.

Saturday, 26 May 2013

Polio [vaccinating] has gone well. We vaccinated 4000 kids more than we vaccinated last month, which was 4000 more than what we had vaccinated previously.

So extrapolating I figure we have about 40,000 more people living in our district compared to last year, and pretty well all of these are Nigerians fleeing violence. For the moment they are mostly staying with relatives of some degree or other, though some have managed to find hovels to rent. Who knows what they are eating or what the strain is and is going to be on the families putting them up.

As violence increased and then later as it became evident that Myra and I were in greater danger, I kept the more worrisome details of our situation out of letters to my family. I had fewer qualms about going into more detail with my younger sister Cora Randall, a professor at the University of Colorado, with whom I had carried on a separate correspondence for many years.

31 May 2013

[e-mail to Cora]

[A] relative calm has taken over since the declaration of the state of emergency [in Borno State, Nigeria] and the sweeping aside of elected officials in favor of the military. I have not been right on the border myself for a long time, but I am told that looking across the road that separates Cameroon from Nigeria in our biggest town, one sees almost no movement—and this in a busy market town that used to be bustling 24 hours a day. Motorcycles are prohibited. The only vehicles are military. People stay indoors. When they must venture out they do so furtively, cautiously, slinking across the dusty roads, for as short a time as possible.

The most recent deaths I have heard about or seen have been assassinations rather than mass shootings or explosions. Yesterday a man and his teenaged daughter were gunned down in their home. Last week a man was stabbed through the heart while sleeping. No robbery involved. Just murder, in and out. Some of these must be revenge killings. Some probably are being done by armed forces personnel in disguise. Some by gang members who suspect a fellow member has betrayed them. Some maybe just for fun…Once killing starts, life becomes cheap. A motorcycle taxi driver from one of our villages was stabbed to death two days ago by his Nigerian passenger who wanted to steal his motorcycle. A used motorcycle here is not worth more than a couple hundred dollars. And for this a family is without a father.

Patients are still arriving from Nigerian villages and towns. I have no idea how they are managing to cross the border.

Monday, 3 June 2013

We are now into the third or fourth week of emergency military rule in Borno State, and it is difficult for anyone here to know what is going on over there. Word on the street is that a lot of ringleaders have been disposed of one way or the other and the more spectacular of the terrorist activities—the bombings, the burnings and the massacres—have abated. There are also however many reports of terrible abuses by the military against innocent civilians. Of course it is impossible to know what is true and what is false, but in times like these it is enough for the public to believe, correctly or not, that abuses are being perpetrated for trouble to ensue. Furthermore, if the spectacular attacks have diminished, assassinations have not, and it is common to get reports of someone (sometimes someone plus a daughter or another family member) being shot to death in his house in the middle of the night. These are vengeance killings or maybe state-sponsored killings or killings in some other way connected to the chaos across the border.

Saturday, 8 June 2013

A baby was born prematurely at home in one of our villages and brought to the nearest health center, whence he was referred on to us. He weighed a kg—2.2 pounds. He was flaccid, ragdoll floppy, a mottled blue color, and as I listened to the mother and watched the baby, I saw him go from a whisper of life to none at all in a matter of seconds. They had not been in my room for even a minute, and one half of my brain was saying, Just let him go, he is obviously too young and too little to survive, given the circumstances of his birth. The other half of my brain was saying, Just do your job, try to bring him back, so what if he doesn't make it. His breathing had stopped completely and so had his heart. There was nothing. The second half of my brain was the one that won out, as it does, and I did CPR—mouth-to-mouth since I had nothing else, this being my office, and neonatal minuscule chest compressions—and once his heart started beating again I gathered him up and ran him down to the delivery room where we have a bag and mask and oxygen. A couple of nurses saw me running and came to my aid. We got him hooked up to the oxygen machine and got the bag and mask going and found a vein through which to inject a bolus of concentrated dextrose. His heart kept going and eventually he started breathing again. By evening he was looking pretty good. We are now 3 days later and all seems to be as it ought to be, so here's hoping.

Day after day he kept breathing, and eventually, although still shy of the two kilograms we usually wanted before discharging our premature babies, this one was hearty enough and his mother was savvy enough that we let him go home. Over the ensuing months we saw him many times in follow-up, and each time he charmed us anew.

As the reliability of our electricity declined steadily, standards slipped, and expectations slipped with them. Complaints and protests were met with blank stares and reports that some districts were going without power for two or three months at a time, so no matter how long the darkness endured, we were told to consider ourselves lucky.

The woman whose face had been burned off would endure darkness forever, but her life was spared, and we did our best to rebuild the integrity of her face. Skin grafts and tiny holes drilled into completely denuded bone coaxed regeneration and nudged healing forward. Her physical stamina and mental health, and those of her mother, who looked after her, left us humbled with awe.

Our Job Is to Take Care of Them to the Best of Our Ability

THE COMMANDANT OF the gendarmerie called me one Thursday evening toward the end of June. He had an emergency and needed my help.

"We've captured four BH in Allagarno. My Land Cruiser's broken down. Can we get the hospital vehicle to go bring them in?"

I called Minista, our driver. He went, and about half an hour later I heard the roar of motors approaching like a freight train up our hill. I looked out the window of my consulting room and saw a posse of motorcycles and some twenty gendarmes and soldiers in bulletproof vests, heavy boots, and black caps. Bands of bullets crisscrossed their waists and chests, and firearms of different sizes and shapes, all of them loud-looking and unambiguous, were clutched in their hands.

I left my office, and by the time I crossed the waiting room and reached the veranda, the captors had dumped three men onto the ground and were furiously kicking and whacking them with their rifle butts. In bellowing voices they informed all three that they were scum. One of the prisoners had a bullet wound in his abdomen. Another, whose pants fell down repeatedly as he rolled or was rolled back and forth on the ground, had two bullet holes in his right leg. The ragged end of that leg's fractured tibia protruded through a third wound.

The commandant explained to me that the three men were from Nigeria and had been sent on an assassination mission, though it was not yet known whom they were being sent to assassinate. Armed with guns and knives, they were stopped at a makeshift checkpoint set up by the gendarmes. Instead of getting out of their car when asked, the would-be assassins opened fire on the gendarmes. There was a skirmish, the intruders were overpowered, and now here they were. A fourth captive had managed to jump out of the pickup and escape.

My job was to administer first aid and do whatever was needed to tack the broken bodies back together. For a reason he did not divulge to me, the commandant had the gendarmes blindfold the injured men while I examined and treated them. None of them had an immediately life-threatening injury, but two needed extensive wound care and suturing, and the broken leg had to be stabilized.

We did all this and gave them shots of penicillin and anti-tetanus serum. As we were finishing, one of the nurses leaned over to me and whispered, "You know,

I'm pretty sure this is all for show. These guys are going to be brought back up to the border, handed over to the Nigerian military, and shot before the night is out."

I mulled this over and conceded. "You might be right," I said, "but our job is to take care of them to the best of our ability as they are, here and now, before us."

The next day as I was timidly protesting the treatment doled out to the prisoners the night before, one of the Cameroonian rapid intervention captains who had been with us said, "You know, we welcome anyone who is fleeing the violence over there and wants to come and live here peacefully. We don't have a problem with that. But they have to come unarmed. If they bring guns, they are coming not to escape war but to make it. We do not want war."

A newspaper article published ten days later claimed that the men had not been handed over to Nigerian authorities after all but had been shipped to Yaoundé "for exploitation."

Wednesday, 26 June 2013

We have six retinoblastoma children on bed with us right now. I don't know what it is about these kids that makes them so irresistible, but they are. You cannot help but love them. Maybe the same is true of all children forced to battle cancer. Our retinos spend on average 4 months with us, so we get to know them and their families. When they come in, the children are miserable. They are scrawny and sick, with no appetite or joy. Then they start treatment and the chemo makes them even more miserable. But if they get through that first cycle, and if they respond to it, as most of them do, slowly but surely they take on new life. For the first time in probably as long as they can remember they are nearly pain-free. They are bald and neither they nor their parents care a twit about that. They charge toward you when they see you coming, smiles stretching from ear to ear. They get the greatest joy out of the simplest things. Most of them come from very far away—Nigeria, the eastern side of Cameroun, [and] one boy on bed right now is from Yaoundé—so they are separated from most of their family. The father of Fatima, a 5 year old girl from Nigeria, who has been with us already for a couple of months, came to visit and brought her a new dress with a sparkly belt and a bright pink head tie, a little doll and a tiny car that runs on batteries, and she has been in seventh heaven for the past week.

On rounds one afternoon I came upon Fatima cowering in a corner, covering her eyes and crying uncontrollably. When I asked her mother what had happened, she replied with resignation that Fatima had been like this all afternoon. "She saw the soldiers," she explained. These were soldiers and gendarmes who had been at the hospital earlier that day to interrogate two gunshot victims we had admitted. Fatima was from Bama, Nigeria, one of the epicenters of BH violence, and a reminder of the horror of whatever she had witnessed there had apparently been triggered by the sight of these uniformed men at the hospital. I wondered how her whole generation of children was going to survive and cope with the atrocities they had seen and been forced to live.

The same day, a middle-aged diabetic man we had followed for years arrived for consultation. He was from a town not far from Fatima's and had always come faithfully to renew his insulin before it finished. This time he was late. He had gone two weeks without an injection, and I asked him why, after he had been so diligent for so long, he had suddenly let his insulin run out. He explained that all the main roads out of Bama were too dangerous for him to travel. I countered that I had been seeing patients from Bama and from towns around Bama every day, so it seemed to me the roads could not be as bad as he thought. He admitted that he had just found out the day before that patients were still getting through. But they weren't coming straight to Kolofata, he said. They were taking long tortuous bush roads to get to us, going west and south before coming east and north, doubling, tripling, and in some cases quadrupling the miles they traversed to reach us.

Sunday, 7 July 2013

There is an American surgeon, a woman, who has expressed interest in coming to work in Kolofata for 6 to 9 months. She seems full of enthusiasm and undaunted by all the things I have had to tell her to dissuade her.

Thursday, 18 July. Yesterday we hosted a day-long visit from a delegation from the U.S. Embassy that included their political attaché, their expert on refugees, their man in charge of security, a translator, four American soldiers (in civilian clothes), and a truckload of Camerounian counterterrorism military personnel as protection. They were here to assess the refugee situation in our corner of the country. We met for an hour and a half and then went to see two groups of recent refugees—one an extended family of 39 and the other a group of 127 people in 8 families that had come over together. As we were sitting down with the second group, a pickup truck loaded with people and pots and pans and mats and sacks rolled into town and the chief pointed and said, See, here comes another one. The stories were all similar. Their town had become a battlefield between Nigerian government forces and extremist forces. Whole neighborhoods were being shot up indiscriminately or burned, and one night as they saw the destruction coming closer and closer to their own homes they made the split-second decision to leave. They gathered up their families and with the clothes on their backs and whatever they could carry in their arms they just left, some on foot, some on bicycle, the lucky ones on motorcycles. Once they got far enough out of town they found trucks or pickups or cars and drivers willing for a price to pick their way through bush paths and [drive] over the border. They were surviving now thanks to the hospitality and generosity of the people of Kolofata, but their fervent hope was to find land and a place of their own and get on with their lives. They had no interest in returning to Nigeria, and no reason to either—they all assumed their homes and possessions were either burned to the ground or thoroughly looted by now.

Tues. 30 July. Sunday afternoon we received two victims of a revenge attack— you never know in these things whether the patients we get are the good guys or the bad guys. One was a gunshot wound to the abdomen. The bullet had not penetrated the abdominal cavity so he was easy to handle. The other had been hacked, eventually to death, with a machete. Both hands had been whacked to bits, his left hip had been chopped open, he had multiple skull fractures under a dozen lacerations to his head. He flailed about wildly but not consciously in his agony.

Saturday, 3 Aug. Malaria has gotten off to a wicked start. We transfused three kids in the nick of time today. A fourth died before we could get blood out of the donor. It could be a long hard season. The extra crowding in homes due to our refugees is not going to help.

What Good Fortune We Americans Have Had

Monday, 26 August 2013

We have been three weeks now without water. There are many tricks one must employ to cope with this. Sponge baths, for one. It takes about a quart of water to do a decent full body bath, a little more if you want to wash your hair. The trick to laundry is to not overdo the soap and to wring clothes out as tightly as possible even before the rinse stage. If you time it right you can hang wrung-out clothes on the line outside and let the rain do the rinsing. Empty basins get lined up under the eaves to catch whatever drops come down. No water goes to waste: rinse water left from laundry or bathing is caught in a bucket and used for flushing the toilet. Dishwashing with minimal water is a whole art in itself. Pots are the worst, so you find yourself planning meals that are oil-less, greaseless, and do not stick to pots and pans, spoons and ladles. The best water you save for drinking, but that, even in less precious times, gets thoroughly boiled and filtered before being bottled for consumption. Cleaning things like sinks and toilets and kitchen counters gets pushed even further down the list of priorities, and we won't even talk about floors.

What is taking up half our days is malaria. We are back to transfusing several children every day, juggling convulsing kids, leaning hopefully over comatose others, soothing tear-drenched parents. Astounding, dramatic cases every day. We save most of them, and that is a comfort and relief. But we don't save them all, and each loss is punch-in-the-stomach painful.

Monday, 02 September 2013

Last Wednesday the governor came to Kolofata to meet with local authorities and representatives of the refugees to see what might be done. I was invited to the main meeting. For our local population and for the Cameroun government, the problems are myriad. Most basically, the people of Kolofata cannot go on feeding all these newcomers. Reserves of food have been used up, the refugees *have no employment and no land of their own to farm. Houses are overcrowded, rents have risen. The government's main concern is that it doesn't know who all these people are. Some, probably most, are legitimate refugees whose homes have been destroyed or rendered too dangerous to return to, but everyone knows that there are also bad guys in the mix—men here either to flee the law or to establish a rear guard or camp from which to launch new strikes or perhaps to extend their crusade throughout northern Cameroun. The United Nations High Commission for Refugees has opened a refugee camp a couple hundred km south of us, and a UNHCR rep was at this meeting pleading with the authorities and the refugees to get the newcomers registered properly and the genuine refugees among them moved into that camp. The local authorities profess to wanting exactly that—Kolofata does not want to go on feeding [them], and we are as concerned as anyone that there might be ill-intentioned elements among them—but the red tape involved in rounding them up and moving them out is horrendous. One can assume that the UNHCR does not want a terrorist cell incubating in their midst either.*

What incredible, extra extraordinary good fortune we Americans have had, to never have known this kind of horror and upheaval.

And now there is talk [in the United States] of mounting a military offensive against the Syrian regime. I understand the rationale, or at least I think I do, but the idea of fighting violence with violence grates. It is primitive and you would think we would be smart enough and clever enough to figure out a better way.

We got the green light for our American surgeon at long last. Of her "6 to 9 months" of availability we lost at least three with the Ministry of Health's foot dragging. We'll see how things go from here.

Thurs. 12 Sept. This is the first year since 2001 that 9/11 came and went without it occurring to me what day it was. It is sad to think of the families and friends for whom that will never happen.

By the end of September, Cameroon had started cracking down on suspicious-seeming or illegal foreigners, and we were told that refugees had started to filter back to Nigeria. We did not see the effects of this reverse movement at the hospital, however, perhaps because as old refugees straggled back west, they did not stay long or else new ones drifted east to take their place.

Myra and I were still being shadowed at all times by gendarmes, so we understood that the government did not believe that victory was at hand.

Our guards were particularly perturbed whenever I was called after hours and obliged to rush up to the hospital in the middle of the night. One day an official visiting from Yaoundé begged me to stop going out at night. I was stunned by this and could only wonder what exactly he thought doctors did. Firemen go where the fire is, soldiers go where the shooting is, doctors go where the sick are. I told him that I had to respond when I was called, and I reminded him that I was always accompanied by armed gendarmes. This, I imagine, was precisely the crux of his concern, though he did not say it. I, too, was painfully aware that every time I went out I was exposing not only myself but the men who went with me, and I wrestled with the wisdom of this, but the people I was being called to assist, lives already known to be at real as opposed to theoretical risk, always won out.

Much of the problem was the season. Malaria was running rampant and the hospital was overrun with children, a third of them suffering malaria-induced encephalitis or severe anemia. Children were admitted two or three to a bed in the pediatric ward, they filled our beds in the overflow ward, and the overflow of the overflow took up space in the adult and even surgical wards. In addition, September was the last month before the new harvest, so malnutrition was at its peak. The combination of malaria and malnutrition was disproportionately more miserable and more deadly than either alone.

Monday, 23 September 2013

We were told that Maiduguri—the capital of Borno State and of the Kanuri tribe, and the city where all the chaos started—has settled down and is back to normal. The grandmother of one of our retinoblastoma patients is from there and she made a three-day visit back home last week. When she returned to Kolofata I asked her how things were there, were they really back to normal as people are saying?

Grandmother: Oh yes, completely normal, everything is fine now.
Me: That's great news. Children are back in school?
Grandmother (hesitantly): Oh, well, no. There are no schools. The schools have been destroyed.
Me: Ah. Are they allowing motorcycles in the streets again?
Grandmother: Oh, well, no. Motorcycles are forbidden because you know they are used for these drive-by shootings.
Me: Then how are people getting around, how do they go to work?
Grandmother: They have to take bicycles, or they take bicycle taxis like in India.
Me: And the phones—are the phones working again?
Grandmother: Oh, well, no, no phones. These terrorists, you know, use phones to make plans, so the government has shut down all the phone lines.
Me: What of the markets? Are the markets open again?
Grandmother: Oh, yes yes, the markets are open everywhere. (Long pause.) But people will not go to them. Nobody will go to them. They are afraid.
Me: Are there foreigners? Do you see Europeans?
Grandmother: Oh yes. Some. A few, I think. But no Chinese. The Chinese have all been killed. Or else they have run away.

So bottom line—Maiduguri doesn't sound to me like it's back to normal. To get there you still have to take a round-about route, going first west and south to get eventually east and north.

Sunday, 13 October 2013

Wednesday we had a 27 year old, 6-month pregnant woman come in with rabies. She had been bitten in August by a dog that died two days later. She had gone to her local health center and been advised to buy anti-rabies vaccine, but this is expensive and the family opted to forego the expense. She started getting a little jittery on Monday, and by the time she reached us she was full-blown rabid, with classic hydrophobia. I have told you before what an awful death rabies is. That state of hyper-hyper-hyper anxiety. They can't swallow anything and so are excruciatingly thirsty. They can't sleep. They are overcome with spastic jitters. They cry out hoarsely in agony. Mentally they remain fully conscious, alert, not benefiting from the "comfort" of coma that comes with other brain diseases. This goes on relentlessly for four or five days, and finally, blessedly, they die.

On the day she came to us, I took the family aside and explained this to them, told them that no matter what, she was going to die and they could either take her home or keep her with us and we would do our best to lessen the awfulness of her death. Many families choose not to waste money on someone who is going to die anyway, but this one decided they would stay. We hospitalized her in a private room and put her on IVs to keep her hydrated so as to reduce the suffering of thirst and bombarded her with diazepam (Valium) and tramadol (a strong injectable analgesic that also dulls the senses), and although it took two days for her to die, those two days were not as terrible as they might have been.

How Do You Say No if the Person Asking Is Holding an AK-47?

COMING HOME FROM a meeting in Maroua, I received a call from an officer named Doni at the American Embassy. She wished to inform me that a new specific and credible threat had been issued, and we were again being targeted for kidnapping. Myra received a call from her embassy as well. The Kolofata commandant came to see us when we arrived back in Kolofata. He stated that his hierarchy was concerned about our safety and sent him to come see how we are doing. We thanked them all.

On October 29, the defense attaché from the US Embassy, Navy Commander John Scudi, came to Kolofata with a team of US and Cameroon military, including Major Kwene, the bright and energetic Cameroonian officer in charge of intelligence in Maroua. (Major—later Colonel—Kwene would be killed by a Boko Haram IED in February 2016.) The senior officers sat with Myra and me in our small meeting room, and we chatted for an hour while the lower ranking

American and Cameroonian troops stood guard around the compound outside. Commander Scudi wanted to know what we thought of the situation and how we were coping. He asked us who we would call if we felt an immediate threat. Major Kwene emphasized that our kidnapping would create a political and diplomatic scandal for the Cameroon government, and that was the main reason he was determined to keep us from harm. He advised us to arrange a safe room at the hospital and another at the house, some corner that could be barricaded from the inside and stocked with a little water and food. If the BH came for us, Major Kwene explained, we were not likely to have time to get to a hideout, but should we be lucky, it would be nice to have that option.

After the meeting, during which we also learned that no one thought the crisis was going to end soon, Commander Scudi took me out of earshot of the others and asked if I would be willing to sign a waiver allowing the NSA to track my telephone. "In case anything happens, it might make it easier for us to find you, and also we can keep track of your calls, see if anything unusual is happening," he explained. I signed the waiver. He followed me into my office, took apart my phone, and wrote down a series of numbers.

> *Wednesday, 30 Oct. We are still struggling with the dearth/lack of anti-retrovirals for our AIDS patients and of antivenin for our snakebites. Our latest snakebite was a woman 7 months pregnant. The snakebite provoked bleeding from her gums and sent her into premature labor. Women in premature labor often bleed a lot anyway, but in this case she was bleeding and unable to clot. Miraculously, by giving her just part of one of our few remaining vials of serum, transfusing her, completing the delivery and praying, we got her stabilized, the bleeding stopped and her life saved. It infuriates me that the antivenin company has been giving us such a hard time, making it impossible for us to get the stuff.*

Being accompanied always by armed guards was a constant reminder of the threat before us, and I discovered that even as I went about my routine work and was absorbed in the problems of the moment, there were certain things I noticed and worried about more as a result of the threat. A car or a motorcycle pulling up or coming the other way on the road set my nerves on edge, made me feel like a dog or a rabbit whose ears perk up at the slightest scent of danger. I could not bear, and so refused, to think of any of the awful things that might follow a kidnapping—the rape, torture, death, my family's distress—so I let my mind concentrate on the ridiculous and mundane: the chances of being abducted with a full bladder, the discomfort of living in the same dress for however many months, getting malaria and having no medicines to treat it. How would I survive without lip balm? Should I be preparing my mind for the long days and months in captivity? How? Upon waking up every morning, the first thought that surfaced to consciousness became, invariably, "Ha! Another night they didn't get me."

31 October 2013

[e-mail to Cora]

The latest activity has been the burning of entire villages along our border—the other side. One of the most recently burned is a twin of one of our own—only meters separating the two. These villages are being burned by what appear to be gangs of vigilantes, but it is widely believed that the gangs are in cahoots with Nigerian government forces. I asked one group of refugee women why someone would want to burn down their village. After a long period of inexact murmuring that amounted to "we have no idea," one woman finally mumbled, "because we let them eat with us," "them" meaning the extremists. Whatever his/her sympathies may or may not be, I'm not sure how anyone is going to say, No, you can't eat with us, if the person doing the asking is holding an AK-47.

Meanwhile we were made aware about three weeks ago that we have been cited anew as targets "by the highest level of leadership" of the wackier wing of the band of bad guys. "Specific and credible," as they say, and "we are taking it very seriously," they say, and this does not make for excessively peaceful peace of mind. (So it is just as well to be drowning, whether in [vaccination] campaigns or patients or anything else, for at least this keeps us focused.) The US and Canadian embassies have been keeping tabs on us again.

The upshot of all this is disappointment, because we had been under the impression that maybe things were easing, at least insofar as our own insecurity was concerned, whereas in fact it seems that for the time being it is the opposite. We remain shackled to our gendarmes.

Meanwhile, our two children's wards are an ocean of kids—two or three to a bed, assorted others all over the floor. Malaria, malnutrition. AIDS and complications of pregnancy in the adult female ward. Trauma and various organ failures in the adult male ward. Tasha [Marenbach], our surgeon, has taken charge of 36 of our 120 beds, and this is a huge help, but getting through the rest still seems to take me forever. And most of our patients are so sick. I rejoice when I come upon a nice one-sickness case like pneumonia or dysentery or tuberculosis. Most patients have a complex combination of intertwining pathologies going on at the same time and would normally require much more time than I have to give them.

Friday, 8 Nov. 2013

Tasha has been working happily away, saving lives that would have been lost had she not been here. I do not understand why every surgeon in the world does not want to do this, at least for a year or two. They should be knocking down our door trying to get in! Among our latest cases are a 14 year old boy with an injury-related deep, pus-filled infection of his right thigh bone, a 30 year old patient with tuberculosis who gave himself a pneumothorax—basically in coughing [he] blew out a lung—and a 40 year old man with gallstones. Next week she will do an elective C-section on one of our promoters.

At dawn on the fourteenth of November, a friend called from Maroua and informed me that during the night Father Georges Vandenbeusch, a forty-two-year-old Parisian priest stationed in Nguetchewe, about thirty kilometers southwest of Kolofata, had been kidnapped from his home. The same day, Lieutenant Colonel Ojong Ojong, the commander of the Thirty-Second Motorized Infantry Battalion in Mora came to see me at the hospital. He was a big fullback of a man wearing a bulletproof vest and carrying a pair of mammoth binoculars around his neck. He said he had come to remind us that our safety was of paramount importance, the work we were doing was essential, everything possible was being done to keep us safe, and we should not be frightened by the events of the night before. Later Amadou Ali called. "*Comment va le moral?*" he asked. We assured him that *le moral* so far was just fine.

Thursday, 28 Nov. 2013

Happy Thanksgiving! Yesterday at around 4 PM, as I was thinking about wrapping up and getting out a bit earlier than usual, for I was tired from the work the night before, a first-time pregnant woman was brought in, referred from one of our health centers. If she was referred, it meant there was a problem, and my heart fell a notch. I let the nurses take the history and do the initial physical exam, and they came with their report: the baby was alive (good) and the woman was stable (good) but she was hypertensive (bad) and bleeding (bad) and short (bad), her cervix was stuck at the same diameter it had been in the health center (bad) and the pelvis was narrow, the baby was big, and it didn't look like there was any way he was going to get out by that route (bad, bad, bad). I went to see for myself, and the nurses were right on all counts except one— the cervix in fact was dilating and looked like it would dilate completely in an hour or so. But the baby's head was so stuck that the separate bones of his skull were overlapping each other. I explained to the family that a C-section was the best solution, and to save the baby it had to be done immediately. The husband turned his pockets inside out to show me he hadn't a franc. They had come on a motorcycle so we told them we would take the motorcycle and lock it up, keep it in hock until he could bring money. The motorcycle was borrowed, he said, and he couldn't do that. I said we didn't care if it was borrowed. I had to go off for a few minutes to tend to another patient and while I was gone one of the husband's comrades hopped on the motorcycle and sped off—removing that payment option. I get so mad at these men who know for 9 months that their wives are pregnant and who do zippo to prepare for any possible complication. Not a franc. They just assume that God—or we, and sometimes I think they confuse the two—will take care of everything. I finished up my afternoon rounds and by the time I got back to the delivery room she was fully dilated. With little hope for success, I got out the vacuum and we had a go. From the first tug I realized that we would succeed. It took six more contractions and a generous episiotomy, and the baby's head came out looking like that tower in Kuala Lumpur, but it did come out, and the rest of the baby did too, and all ended with smiles (us) and furious wails (the little guy).

Monday, 9 December 2013

After all was over I talked to this man [the husband of the woman in the last letter], asked him why he had not at least put a little aside each month for nine months so that, should anything go wrong at the end, he would be able to handle it. He looked at me as if the answer to that were so obvious it was not even worth speaking, and then he said, "If I had money like that on hand it would be too tempting and I would spend it on something else first." So better not to have it. The logic is brilliant.

Our latest polio campaign went well, as we vaccinated over 48,000 under-fives. We figure about 11,000 or 12,000 of those are refugees or newcomers. There was fighting over the border the first day and night so our teams were hampered at first—we pulled them back for fear of getting hit by stray bullets, not because there was any shooting being done on our side—but they were able to go back on Saturday and Sunday and get the coverage we had hoped for. This campaign was our 6th for 2013. And yet polio is increasing in some places and coming back in places it had not been for years, like in the south of Cameroon, and now I see there have been several cases found in Syria. I am not saying that the fight against polio is a hopeless endeavor, but I think anyone with an open mind can see that this is not the best way of waging it.

Wednesday, 11 Dec. Monday and Tuesday Kolofata played host to a big regional meeting, presided by the governor, to discuss security issues. There were about 80 people involved, many of them men in different colored uniforms—blue, green, camouflage, khaki—with varying amounts of gold bars and glitter on their chests and shoulders. Yesterday afternoon to close the event the governor hosted a dinner at the sous-préfet's. We were stunned and discomfited when in his pre-dinner speech the governor started to go on at length thanking us for being here and for having stayed when other foreigners, one nationality after the other, left in the wake of the events of last February, taking with them their expertise, their service and their funds. He spelled out to the assembled glitter and boffins why it is important that we be protected and, looking directly at us, said, "You may not see me, but rest assured I see you, and I am with you every day." This took us by surprise and had me squirming inside while wondering what was the underlying message, the hidden agenda, the politics behind the torrent of words.

Trekking to Go Somewhere, Anywhere

Monday, 30 December 2013

We have had no shortages of trauma victims over the holidays, but only one or maybe two related to the goings-on in Nigeria. The one we are sure of is a young man who caught a piece of shrapnel in his abdomen. It pierced his intestine so *he came in with what amounted to a battle-induced colostomy. He said a bomb was dropped on their compound, killing his father instantly. He looked up and found his father without a face. It is not clear that the son is going to live either but we dare to hope. Tasha's skills and daring are being tested to the limit.*

After being in Boko Haram captivity for a month and a half, Father Georges Vandenbeusch was liberated "for compassionate reasons." He dismissed this, scoffing, "These people have compassion for no one."

Wednesday, 8 January 2014

Unusual for this time of year, the electricity has been very unstable. There have been no rainstorms to knock power lines down, wind storms have not started yet. No ice storms either. Just no power, and no explanation. This does not auger well for the upcoming rainy season. I think we should mentally prepare now for total blackout. A number of years ago during a spree of privatization of state companies, a big American firm, AES, bought a majority stake in Cameroon's electricity company. We were so optimistic. At last, we were going to get a more reliable power supply, breakdowns were going to be fixed more quickly or avoided altogether. In spite of an early publicity campaign involving American-styled brochures ("We are your new electricity supply country, we are here to serve you," etc.) and even polite apologetic notices sent around to bigger customers and essential services in advance of a scheduled power outage, things rapidly went from bad to worse to unbelievable. The cheery brochures disappeared. Within months the company gave up advising us in advance of power cuts, I assume because there were so many unscheduled cuts that it was ridiculous to bother to point out the scheduled ones. And prolonged outages of days, then weeks, wore us all down until we stopped complaining to them, recognizing the futility of it. Rumor has it now that AES is throwing up its hands, looking to get out, and buyers are not exactly lining up around the block.

It was quarter past six, and we had just finished breakfast on the morning of January 15 when we heard the first boom. I thought it must be a truck backfiring, or maybe a large metal gate slamming. But then there was a second and then a third boom, and I began to doubt that it was anything but the sounds of bombardment. We went up to the hospital, and all through rounds, through the morning and into the afternoon, the booms continued. They shook our buildings so hard we could hear the metal roofs rattle.

The Nigerian government was on the offensive. Along the border on both sides villages were being hit by artillery fire on the ground and bombs from the air. We could stand on our hill and see the planes. Excited rumor had it that one was being piloted by a woman.

Whether the villages on the Cameroon side of the border were being hit by accident or intention depended on who was asked. No one denied that Boko Haram militants from Nigeria took refuge in Cameroon. Opinion differed on whether they were also using Cameroon as a rear base of operations and a recruiting ground for future militants.

Cameroon's government was in a terrible bind. It did not want the country to be used as either a rear base or a recruiting ground, but it also did not want to turn on its own citizens. Distinguishing a Cameroonian from a Nigerian was almost impossible, since for years, through a mix of bribery and trickery, thousands of Nigerians, evidently anticipating events that would unfold, contrived to procure Cameroonian identification cards—vital proof of nationality. When trouble started, Nigerians fleeing their own country came to stay with relatives in Cameroon, where they were so well hidden and protected that when the time came to track down terrorists who undertook actions in Nigeria and then ducked into Cameroon to hide, it was impossible to separate Nigerians from Cameroonians. Hundreds, perhaps thousands, of Nigerians were carrying Cameroonian ID. The Cameroon government could not round up "foreigners" with Cameroonian identification without looking as if they were assailing their own people. Yet if Cameroon didn't round them up, the Nigerian government got angrier and angrier and accused Cameroon of supporting the rebels. If Cameroon did attempt to round them up, Boko Haram threatened to kidnap—and then did kidnap—non-African expats caught in the political cross fire.

The bombing and gunfire continued through Saturday, when an apparent agreement was reached to allow women and children to cross the border. They streamed over, each woman with a cloth bundle balanced on her head, a baby on her back, and a toddler by each hand. They came on foot, all trekking just to go somewhere, anywhere, away.

Cameroonian residents of the larger villages along the border left as well, as even with the cease-fire most believed the violence would begin again sooner rather than later.

We ran a door-to-door polio vaccination campaign that weekend, and for the first time the violence and insecurity prevented us from reaching all of our villages.

Tasha was submerged in trauma cases—open fractures, bullet wounds, shrapnel embedded in a variety of body parts, and burns.

Where I Come from, You Do Not Ask Questions

ON SATURDAY, THE first of February, just before five p.m., I was doing afternoon rounds on hospital beds filled to capacity when Amadou Ali called. He asked how I was, said he was glad to find us still here, and added that Madi Talba, his brother-in-law, was coming to see me with a message. A half hour later we had just parked the Land Rover at home when Madi pulled in and hastened out of his car. He bubbled, "They have declared clearly, they are already taking steps, this time it will happen. They are coming to kidnap you. You have to leave Kolofata— discretely, like while the town is at prayer, so no one notices. Six fifteen, six thirty at the latest, in a vehicle people don't know, not your own. Go to Maroua, stay for two or three days until all the authorities have been informed and measures have been put in place to protect you."

Two thoughts crashed into my mind. First, with the gendarmes we had had around us day and night for the past year, had we not been protected? And second, how could anyone say two or three days would not become two or three weeks, two or three months, forever?

If my Land Rover was out of the question, so was the hospital vehicle. We had a new Toyota pickup that we had purchased a year earlier and then, because of the security situation, kept hidden in a garage. It had been neither used nor seen by anyone but us and Minista, the hospital's driver. I asked Madi if Minista could accompany us, and he agreed. I also reminded him that although we were being told to inform no one, our gendarmes would have to be told; otherwise they would not let us out of our own gate. To this also he agreed. The head gendarme insisted on accompanying us, together with his second in command. Our bags, never unpacked, were ready. We waited until evening prayers had started and then we set out, Myra and I riding the whole way doubled over in the back of the cabin, our heads below window level.

We camped at Amadou Ali's house in Maroua and three days later were informed that it was safe to return to Kolofata. We had no idea and no way of knowing what might have happened had we not left when we did.

15 February 2014

[e-mail to Cora]

It is relatively quiet on the border, though the baseline violence flares occasionally. Every once in a while we hear of a BH being tracked down and killed inside Cameroon. Or a guy suspected of helping the Nigerian military. On the Friday before last the Nigerian military chased a bunch of BH over the border, followed them into Cameroon, and when they caught up with them in one of our villages, the army (Nigerian army, I repeat) opened fire, killing two bad guys but also in the process four innocent Cameroonian civilians, including a 70 year old [man]. These things, which should be plastered all over the media and condemned as intolerable international incidents, do not even make the news here, let alone elsewhere.

A couple of days ago 39 people were killed in another village over the border, a village from which we used to get a lot of patients, and at least 100 homes there were burned to the ground. Threats of kidnapping of foreigners have resurfaced. We continue to be guarded around the clock. (This is ridiculous to say and melodramatic surely, but if the unthinkable were ever to happen I would never forgive myself if I had not said it, so let me go on the record, to you and you alone, and I am absolutely serious about this: if some day that unthinkable were to happen and I were kidnapped, not a penny in ransom is to be paid. Ransom money with these guys goes to buy arms that will kill innocent people and do ever more damage, and no single life is worth that, and definitely mine is not: all I will have lived for up to that point would be irreversibly obliterated. Note that in this I speak for no one but myself.)

Sunday, 16 February 2014

We got back Friday evening from a 3-day Maroua meeting. We were supposed to have gotten back Saturday night, but I refused to waste another day listening to drivel and left my nurse behind to finish up the last day. They had heard enough from me anyway. I try my best to be polite and as Camerounian as I can be, but I'm sure the presenters, presiders and participants cringe when my hand goes up.

Friday night there were a number of catastrophes awaiting and yesterday and today have so far been full of emergencies, accidents, complicated pregnancies, and patients in dire straits. The two worst cases were women hemorrhaging.

Of Saturday's cases, one was a young man whacked with a machete, sent to us from a hospital in Nigeria. His left wrist was hacked, but the worst injury was to his head. His assailant must have tried to decapitate him and he, our patient, must have ducked. The whole top of his scalp, down to the bone, which was also scraped, was sliced off. He looked like a monk, except instead of the top of his head just being shaved, it was missing. Tasha spent six hours in the O.R. putting him back together. Another young man came in yesterday. This one, a nurse in a Nigerian hospital just over the border, [had] been on a motorcycle when it collided with another one. His face was smashed on the left side and he was seeing stars. Terrific headache this morning but should be okay.

As I write—midday Sunday—Tasha is operating on a 10 year old boy [who] fell out of a tree 6 days ago. In Nigeria. They only made their way to us last night. He was in a dreadful state. I am not sure what is ruptured in his abdomen, but he was in terrible pain, his abdomen distended with fluid—probably some combination of blood, pus and stool. Difficulty breathing because the distended abdomen was pressing up against his diaphragm. Dehydrated. Hypoxic. Anemic. We spent the night trying to get him up to some minimal operable state. Upon opening him up, Tasha found a fracture of the boy's pelvis and the bladder and several loops of intestine pierced by the jagged edge of the broken bone. She spent four hours on him in the O.R. and he survived that and now we will wait and see. We hope his guardian angel is back on the job making up for lost time.

February 2014

[e-mail to Jackie French, a friend]

Things have been relatively calm here since the border bombardments of three weeks ago. Isolated incidents, but that's all. Once more we are tempted to feel hopeful. I don't remember if I told you that the new head of the Nigerian military stated publicly that by April the terrorism problems in northeast Nigeria would be over. We are looking forward to April and hope that Nigeria's problems do not end because all the bad guys are taking refuge in Cameroon!

Thursday, 27 February 2014

Myra is off to Maroua to get us some anti-snake serum, the stuff we have been trying to get our hands on for the past year, unsuccessfully. There is only one company in the world that makes it, Sanofi-Pasteur in France, and it has been out of production for [a] year. We were finally told that we could get 30 doses. Then they knocked that down to 15. It stands now at 10, and we will have to be satisfied with that. We have long since stopped giving full doses to patients and find we can manage them fine giving only half or even sometimes 1/3 doses so long as we keep them on strict bed rest for a week. So we will stretch these 10 doses out to save 20 or 25 patients, and in that way we will hold on a little while longer.

I told you in my last letter about the 10 year old boy [with] a broken pelvis and both the urinary bladder and the intestine torn open by a jagged end of bone. Clearly the boy had suffered some violent trauma. Pre-operatively, when he first brought his son in, the father had been vague, spoke of the boy complaining of "stomach pains." Only when specifically asked about trauma did he relate that his son had said something about having fallen out of a tree while playing with his friends. "Falling out of a tree" is the local equivalent of the U.S. housewife's "tripping on a stair" to explain the bruises of spouse abuse. Except here it is not usually family abuse that is being hidden but rather some crime and even though the patient may be the victim there is often little desire to get caught up in the tangled nets of the forces of law and order. After the surgery, when we realized the extent of the boy's injuries, we took the father aside and tried to get a clearer history from him. As it turned out, they were not even from the village they initially claimed they were from but rather from another town that has been viciously attacked recently on at least two occasions. A Nigerian town of course. A hotbed of extremism and unrest. Apart from that admission, the father's tale shed no further light on what happened to his son. At first the boy fell out of a tree, then a tree fell on the boy, then he really had no idea what had happened to his son. The father had been away from home and when he came back in the afternoon he found that "someone" had brought his son back to the house like that. No, he didn't know who had brought him, no it hadn't occurred to him to try to find out, no he didn't know what had happened, no he didn't know who the boy had been with. "Where I come from," he said simply, "you do not ask questions."

2 March 2014

[e-mail to Cora]

Nothing has abated in Nigeria. Three days ago the BH attacked a secondary school in Yobe State and killed 43 sleeping students. It was the third or fourth major attack on a school in the North in recent months. Last night one of our own border villages had two mortars fired at it (I saw the munitions they found, as a policeman brought them in this morning, big spiky club-like things) and a woman in the same village reputed to be sleeping with a Nigerian soldier had her throat slit. Every week or so I have been getting calls or visits warning us with varying degrees of urgency to be prudent, the bad guys are reconnoitering and planning to snatch us away, and we listen to these things and just never know what to think of them. The Nigerian government appears to be inappropriately indifferent to the plight of the North [and] refuses to ask for outside help.

5 March 2014

[e-mail to Cora, in response to articles she sent]

Very good articles, both of them. Just a couple of comments. The one guy who talks about BH consisting of "a few hundred men hiding out" is way off the mark, unfortunately. Intelligence reports talk of 12000 BH fighters inhabiting one forest alone not too far from here, and there have to be thousands more scattered throughout towns and cities. The leadership is known to have ties with better known groups whose names I will not write. It is sickeningly true that the Nigerian military is doing virtually nothing to prevent or stop the attacks. They either cower in their barracks when something happens nearby or they literally run away. Military bases have been targeted as well, and seemingly at will. The governor of Borno State was courageous and took his life in his hands when he finally said publicly that the military situation was a disgrace, that the terrorists are better armed, equipped and manned than the Nigerian army, and that as things stand now there is no way this war against terrorism in the north can be won. The President of Nigeria, [who] responded to this by saying peevishly that in that case he would consider withdrawing all the military from the north and seeing how the governor fares without them, appears to be an idiot.

We Wondered if Kolofata Was Being Set Up as the Bull's-Eye

Friday, 14 March 2014

We are looking at the possibility of having to close our health center in Amchide, on the border with Nigeria, given the increase in violence on the other side and the increased spillage of that violence onto our side. The nurses working there have become more and more anxious—and less and less present at work. Following rumors that public edifices were going to be attacked and burned down (the health center being a public edifice), much of the town's population fled and whole neighborhoods remain virtually uninhabited. I made plans on Tuesday to go up there the following day, have a meeting with the nurses and *other personnel, but at ten p.m. I started getting a barrage of phone calls—the mayor, the* sous-préfet, *eventually AA—from people all telling me they "had heard" that I was planning to go to Amchide the next day and informing me that it was out of the question. Period.*

Myra got a call from the Canadian High Commission. Out of the blue, no particular reason, just checking up. And this afternoon I got a call from the governor. Same thing. Out of the blue, no particular reason, or at least none that he stated.

18 March 2014

[e-mail to Cora]

Things are getting worse. More grenades, mortars, stray bullets [are] finding their way over "by accident." It is getting harder to believe the accident part. The current thinking is that the Nigerian government, or at least the Nigerian army, is hoping to provoke Cameroon into responding. I am not sure which response they are hoping for: a greater Cameroonian effort to round up the BH, or an armed riposte against those (the Nigerian army) who are "accidentally" lobbing munitions against us. If the latter, one would suppose the idea in their heads is to give Nigeria the "right" to invade Russian-style, maybe lop off this part of Cameroon so that they themselves can grab the BH hiding out here. If the former, Cameroon catching and locking up more BH would put foreigners up here, the few of us who are left, at even higher risk of kidnapping. Cameroon's official policy is to maintain peace at all costs, and so, to reduce the likelihood of a rogue (or drunk) member of our armed forces at the border responding to these provocations, the men have been recalled to barracks and no longer patrol the vulnerable border areas as before. This leaves the populations of those towns ever more exposed, and in places there has been such panic that whole towns have emptied of their populations.

Friday, 28 March 2014

The most recent wild delivery was a woman in labor with her 6th child, who by the time she came to us was already dead—the baby, not the mother. The baby was huge, which for a 6th delivery should not have posed much of a problem, but he was also badly positioned, and that did. I hate to resort to C-section for dead babies, so we set about trying to deliver her vaginally. It took us nearly an hour of pulling with the vacuum to get the massive head out and then reaching in to get the body turned so we could haul the shoulders out, first one, then the other, and by the time we finished my back felt like it had been stretched on a rack, my shoulders like they had been pummeled, my forearms like they had been run over by a heavy vehicle, and my fingers like they had been caught in a slammed door. The mother, when it was over, was cool as a cucumber and looked about as tired as she might be after a particularly arduous shopping expedition. She was so delighted to get that baby born. She is from quite far away inside Nigeria, so she is staying with us for the week until she can get her episiotomy sutures out. Any time I go by her bed, she lights up with the most beautiful smile.

29 March 2014

[e-mail to Cora]

On Wednesday—or was it Thursday?—morning, the Nigerian army went on the rampage hunting down some BH on the border. In their zeal, the military came onto our side, guns blazing. The head nurse in our health center there called me to tell me. I told him to make sure all our nurses were in the health center and that they stayed hunkered down inside until the shooting stopped. He assured me he was doing that. Our other health center 5 km down the road called to say they were sending two victims, a woman and a 12 year old girl. Both patients arrived about half an hour later, but for the girl it was too late. She had been shot in the abdomen—her intestines were outside her body—and died before we could get her onto the operating table. The woman fared better. She had been shot in the left hand. Severed some tendons and crushed some bones. We don't know whether these two were caught in the cross fire or if they were deliberately shot. When the BH want to settle a score, they have a reputation for taking their anger out on daughters or wives of the men they wish to punish, so it is not inconceivable that these two were targeted.

Thursday night I was called to see a comatose man with a high fever and while I was seeing him, an army truck pulled up and the helmeted, bulletproof-vested soldiers dragged out onto the ground a young man tied up and on a leash. The man smelled of stool—he had defecated into his pants—and his head and face were covered with blood. The story was that he and three of his companions (all Nigerians, presumably BH) had been in one of our villages on the border flaunting videos of women and children getting their throats slit. [The young men had been] claiming that they were the ones doing the slitting. The military got wind of this and raided the village, seized the men and their phones, loaded them into the truck and were bringing them to Kolofata when the one who ended up being our patient jumped out of the truck—some said in an effort to escape, others said in an effort to commit suicide by throwing himself under the wheels of the truck. In any case, all he succeeded in doing was splitting open his scalp and scraping up his arms and legs. We cleaned his wounds, stitched him up, and sent him back into the keeping of the soldiers, wishing him abundant good luck.

6 April 2014

[e-mail to Cora]

On Friday evening I was called by one of our health workers on the border. He reported that the town there was in a state of panic, as a group of Cameroonian soldiers had uncovered a stash of BH cash (to be used for buying arms, presumably), arrested the culpable and, since the culpable were Nigerian, turned them over to their military counterparts on the other side of the border. As was to be expected, and as I later learned to be the case, these men were executed on the spot. Reprisals en masse were feared, and so the Cameroon side of the town was emptying of its population, people anticipating the worst and fleeing to avoid it. What was not clear was whether the reprisals were being planned because these guys had been turned over for certain execution or whether it was because the Cameroonians involved were being accused of having stolen the loot.

The local authorities panicked as well. Some here in Kolofata gathered up their wives and children and shipped them to safer territory away from the border. We were contacted late Friday evening and advised to get out of town. At that point M and I both considered that going off into the night was more of a risk than staying put, so we stayed put.

At five o'clock the next morning, our friend from Maroua called again. Hearing her voice, I expected bad news. She apologized for the hour and then said she thought we should know, in case we wanted to leave Kolofata for a while, that two Italian priests and a Canadian nun had been kidnapped in the night from their mission compound in Tchere, a town on the main road between Kolofata and Maroua. Gangs of armed men on motorcycles had done the snatching.

The Canadian High Commission called a little later. The nun was old and battling cancer. She had been in Cameroon for over thirty years and had been due to return to Canada the following week.

It occurred to us that now there had been expatriates kidnapped from villages to the northeast, to the southwest, and to the southeast of us. We wondered if they were tiptoeing around us, or if Kolofata was being set up as the bull's-eye.

Our reason for not leaving remained simple: we did not want to hand the enemy such an easy victory. They could dismantle the infrastructure of northern Cameroon cheaply and painlessly, piece by piece, if by just issuing threats they could have others do their bidding. It seemed to us that a great deal of courage was going to be demanded of the people of our district over the months ahead, and this did not seem to be a good time for any of us to show fear.

It was peculiar to live knowing that on any day or night I could be sought out, set upon, kidnapped, and bundled off to a place like northern Nigeria at a time when it was waging ruthless war with itself. If not killed outright, I wondered if I would be psychologically and physically sturdy enough to survive the ordeal. I feared the grief a kidnapping would cause my family and the trouble it would cause my government. I did not want to be stupid or reckless, and maybe staying was both, but I also asked myself constantly which was more stupid: to stay in defiance of sensible advice or to be cowed by a threat and run away, leaving others behind to cope? And which was more reckless: to disregard an alleged danger or to abandon all those whose trust had been not easily won but who trusted us now, who relied on us, and who in the difficult days to come might have to rely on us more than ever?

Myra and I realized we were the only foreigners left in our part of the country, but if the BH did come for us, we also realized that our kidnapping would not be the last. They would come for others after us—children of the wealthy, government officials, village chiefs—and then there would be no end. We did not imagine that our work accorded us any protection; on the contrary, it was evident that with our white skin and North American sympathizers we would be seen as a prize. The start of our biennial leave was due for the end of June, and we reaffirmed our decision to stay until then. We hoped that by the time that three-month break was over, some measure of normalcy would have returned.

Not Longer Than Seven Years, Seven Weeks, and Seven Days

Monday, 14 April 2014

I took a thermometer outside yesterday. It was an overcast day, sun filtering through a thin layer of stratus clouds, but I found a nice shady spot under a clump of trees. I left the thermometer there for a while to cool down, and it got to 117 degrees, just to give you an indication. It's a tough time to be without water.

Tuesday, 15 April. Still no electricity. It tried to come on for about 30 seconds yesterday evening (how hope soars!) but then poof. Someone did not get his A connected to his B quite right. We will see what today brings.

There was more unrest [in Amchide] Sunday and yesterday. A policeman and a gendarme were shot in a drive-by (motorcycle) shooting. Neither died, but the fact that it happened is worrisome and it got up the ire of the armed forces who the next day carried out a massive door-to-door search in Amchide, looking for arms or suspicious characters. I am told that five people were killed in the exercise. Over the weekend there was more firing just on the other side of the border, and yesterday a bomb attack on a crowded bus station near Abuja, Nigeria's capital, that killed close to 100 people according to initial reports. All the lip service offered by political leaders about taking control and putting an end to the chaos appears to be only that.

Sunday, 20 April 2014

AA came into town Friday around noon and left 24 hours later. It is interesting to hear his views on the current situation. At one point Myra asked him how long he thought it would last and how he thought it would end. He replied that in Kanuri tradition, conflicts of this sort cannot last longer than seven years, seven weeks and seven days. That was the length of time it took to defeat the last great conqueror of the Kanuris. (The difference this time being that to a large extent it is Kanuris attacking Kanuris…) So, he said, since BH started its activities in 2009, we only had, at most, 2 years left. And they would surely be defeated. So he pronounced. And so we will see.

20 April 2014

[e-mail to Cora]

AA seems to be frustrated above all by the Nigerian government's refusal to acknowledge that they are not in the least in control of the situation. He thinks the only way to regain the upper hand is for the Americans, the French and the British to get involved. But the Nigerian government refuses to ask for help, and foreign powers will not get involved without being asked. The Nigerian government does not want to admit that it is not in control. But it is not, and everyone here knows that it is not. And the more the BH get away with their crimes, the more the population will shift to the BH side, in spite of their gruesome acts. People generally just want to be with the winners, justice and honor and ideology be damned, and then to be left alone.

Monday, 05 May 2014

This will not be my last letter to you, but we are counting down. Things are a little more complicated this year than in the past, as for security reasons we cannot tell anyone when we are leaving. All our preparations have to be done surreptitiously and without consultation.

To complicate matters, cholera has turned up in a village 2 districts away from us, in a community of Nigerian refugees. This has been one of our fears.

Wed. 07 May. Thanks to the kidnapping of those 279 girls from a school in [Chibok] Nigeria, our Boko Haram are finally making the news in the rest of the world. It is about time. These guys have been wreaking unspeakable havoc for the past 5 years and the world beyond Nigeria and its immediate neighbors has been all but deaf and blind to it. I guess the question now must be, is all this attention going to make things better or worse? My own feeling is that if the U.S. and Europe really want to do something about it, it is not too late to extinguish the flames relatively quickly. But my fear is that the fighting words coming out of western capitals are just words, political positioning to be followed up by, at most, some ineffectual gesture.

8 May 2014

[e-mail to Cora]

Many among the local population, or at least among that part of it that listens to the news, dare to hope for the best. They have heard that "the Americans are coming" and since everyone knows there is nothing the Americans cannot do, this has to be the beginning of the end. Yet others have the opposite opinion: that getting the attention of the outside world is exactly what the BH have been trying, heretofore unsuccessfully, to do all along; now that they've got it, the brainless thugs will be bringing out the real fireworks, before which all that they have done up to now will pale.

The BH's latest adventures have included the razing of a village on the border, another of Nigeria's villages that used to send us quite a few patients, many of whom I assume are now dead, and the killing of an officer of the Cameroonian gendarmerie when they stormed one of our gendarme posts to free two prisoners.

18 May 2014

[e-mail to Cora]

Friday night ten Chinese men working on reconstructing the road north of Mora were kidnapped when their camp was invaded by the usual crowd from over the border—except this time the invasion was with tanks and artillery, not just a posse on twenty motorcycles. The workers had been guarded by Cameroon's most elite branch of the military, but our soldiers were only 10 or 20 in number with nothing but rifles and sidearms, no match for the hundred or so heavily weaponed men who invaded. It marks the first time that an actual battle was brought by the terrorists onto Cameroon soil, and it has filled the local authorities, not to say all the rest of us, with horror and cold fear. Reports vary, but it would appear that at least one Chinese worker and one Cameroonian soldier were killed in the attack.

One thing living through this time in this place does is make you ecstatic each morning when you wake up and realize you are in your own bed, alive and safe, and that the town is alive and safe, and that there is a whole day of sunlight to look forward to before night falls again.

Whatever You Can Do, You Should Do

WHILE SOME AUTHORITIES were grateful that we had not left and urged us to stay, others felt the danger had grown too great. They did not want an international incident any more than we wanted to be kidnapped, and the decision to stay was one we considered and made anew every day. We were prudent in sticking to home and hospital and felt protected by the men around us, but also, although we realized the hospital would survive our absence, the wish not to diminish the morale of staff and community by disappearing before our scheduled leave date in late June kept us from going.

Tasha also was against going before her planned date of departure, but as a concession to our more anxious authorities and to reduce my own concern, I convinced her to leave a week early. So she was not in Kolofata when at noon on the last Sunday in May the nurse on duty called me to say he had just received a woman at term referred from one of our health centers for massive bleeding. The baby was already dead, the woman was very pale, and the cervix through which the child had to pass was barely dilated.

I asked a few questions of the nurse and determined that it was most likely a case of premature detachment of the placenta. Given that true labor had not yet begun and that the woman was already dangerously anemic, I told him to refer her immediately to Mora or Maroua for surgery.

Two minutes later the nurse called back. "They won't go. They are from Nigeria and they don't have papers. The man says if they try to go any further inside Cameroon, they will be arrested."

I went up and tried to reason with the man, told him I would write a letter explaining the condition of his wife and asking authorities along the way to let him pass. He was not interested.

"Whatever you can do, you should do," he said, and left it at that.

The woman was conscious, but her eyes stared blankly. We got an oxytocin drip to induce labor going into a vein in one arm and a blood transfusion running into the other. We fired up the generator, so she could have some oxygen. We catheterized her and ruptured the amniotic sac. We got a second donor screened and drew his blood.

The cervix dilated just as we told it to. The blood, fluids, and oxygen kept her alive. Within three hours her cervix, still not fully dilated, was wide enough to allow us to get the vacuum cup on the baby's head and to pull him out. The detached placenta followed immediately, along with an ocean of blood—some of it, I was relieved to see, with clots.

She stayed on the table, head lower than her body, for another two hours. A nurse kept a firm grip on her lazy uterus as more blood and fluids poured into her. And then, just like that, she was fine: when it was over, it was over. A hint of pink came back into her conjunctivae. She began to talk. We helped her to sit up. She smiled. I was ecstatic.

Monday, 26 May 2014

We had a good weekend, but boiling hot. The electricity has been out since Friday afternoon so the house has been airless and stifling. There was water for half an hour on Saturday so I managed to get a couple of dresses washed—but that was all I accomplished all weekend. Apart from saving the odd life here and there I mean.

The hot season is mating season for our peacocks, so we have been treated to some dazzling displays. They are not the brightest of creatures—pea brained, one might say—and a few days ago we came upon one, feathers fully flared, prancing and dancing and shaking, courting...our garbage can. Yesterday we came home from the hospital and found one standing right there in our court-yard when we came through the gate, his huge fanned tail magnificent, sparkling in the sunlight. We walked past him and he did not flex a muscle or retreat an inch, just stood there as if to say, Have you ever seen anything so beautiful? There is another peacock—or maybe the same one—that seems to guard our house every night. At about 5:30 each evening he takes up position on the low wall that juts beside my bedroom and he stays there all night. Myra calls him our guardian angel. He may be that. Peacocks make good night guards because they call out at the slightest unexpected noise. Of course, they make bad night guards for the same reason. They call out so often no one pays them the least attention.

Among the Slaughtered Are Many We Cared For

Monday, 2 June 2014

This, then, is my final letter this time around.

Another weekend spent without light or water.

The good news yesterday—I don't think you follow these things, but it was very good news for all of us here—was the freeing of the Canadian nun (74 years old) and the two Italian priests kidnapped by the BH crowd two months ago. They were handed over at the border not far from here and made their way to Yaoundé yesterday.

Last week the Cameroun government deployed a thousand troops—many, or maybe mostly, specially trained commandos and rapid intervention forces—to fortify the border. They lost no time getting to work. There is a new base (all army tents) set up half a mile down from the hospital. They have been carrying out fact-finding missions in several of our villages known to harbor BH sympathizers, and some of these fact-finding missions have been on the brutal side, and there are bodies to prove it. In a few of the more egregious cases, bodies riddled with bullets have been left on the side of the road to rot—as a warning. As one policeman said after witnessing one of these, "I will not be eating meat for a month." We were polio vaccinating this weekend and one of our nurses had to pass by one of these cadavers—intestines hanging out, brain spilling from the skull—to get to her assigned village, and she came back traumatized. "But" I said to her, "you have seen plenty of dead bodies in your time." "Not," she replied, "like this."

I imagine these commandos have already killed some innocent people, and my fear, and I think the fear of many, is that they get kill-crazy and lose the goodwill of the people. So far most people seem to be happy they are here and there is more hope than I have seen since the beginning that maybe we will after all get out of this jungle before it gets any darker.

One highlight of my weekend was yesterday afternoon's delivery of twins. Deliveries are almost always fun, and with twins you get a bonus. This woman had already delivered 8 children (5 alive) and she looked like she was carrying Mount Everest sideways. When I told her on arrival that she was pregnant with twins she said, pointing to her enormous belly, I thought so. She also had an excessive volume of amniotic fluid, so when I went to rupture her membranes,

I knew I had better duck and move to one side—and I did both but neither fast enough. I got drenched and the rest of the day smelled like the seashore after the tide has gone out. Without water I could not wash off [as] lavishly as I would have liked. The twins, both boys, are sturdy and strong and gorgeous.

Thursday, 3 June

As if it was a premonition, my mentioning kill-crazy soldiers, yesterday morning at 8:45 I received a call informing me that one of our nurses had been shot dead in Mora during the night. The story is not clear but it sounds like it involved a combination of the nurse being out on his motorcycle after curfew and a drunk soldier. Four children, pregnant wife.

Not a happy note to end on, but end I must. We have our hands full and will never get done all we have to get done between now and when it all has to get done. But we are forging on, with much anticipation and excitement. Keep fit and well and don't fall. I will see you very soon.

Much, much love,

Ellen

In Nigeria schools were being destroyed and students murdered. Marketplaces and towns were being set ablaze. The villages making news around the world—Damboa, Bama, Banki, Damaturu, Gwoza, Pulka, Tchachile, and so many others—were villages where people considered Kolofata their hospital. I wondered sadly how many of those killed and maimed were lives we once had saved, patients whose sight we had restored, babies who had been born into our hands. Among the slaughtered were smiling, carefree, happy men, women, and children who had done nothing to deserve their savage fate. Our people. I seethed to think of thugs blithely scything them all down like so many stalks of grain.

In Kolofata our streets were now full of soldiers, commandos, rapid intervention forces, gendarmes, even parachutists manning checkpoints, searching homes, and patrolling neighborhoods round the clock.

On June 20 Myra and I left Kolofata as planned. All that had had to be done to facilitate operations and prepare hospital staff for our three-month absence had been done. Then at home we had packed our bags, cleaned out our refrigerators, poured antitermite solution along the cracks of our floors, and covered our furniture with sheets of plastic—all the things we did every two years before our late June departure. We did nothing more than usual, having no reason to think we would not be back in three months.

23 June 2014

[e-mail to Cora]

I will get this off to you under the wire.

We are in Yaoundé as of Friday night, will fly to Paris tonight.

Last night we learned that there was an attack on a military outpost at one of our border villages; as we went to bed around eleven we still did not know whether it was over or what the outcome was, but some military casualties had started to arrive at the hospital. This morning phone calls are not getting through to Kolofata, so we are frustrated and on edge.

Have a good day and a good week, and I'll be talking to you soon.

Love,

Ellen

Epilogue

FIVE WEEKS LATER, Boko Haram attacked Kolofata. Buildings and vehicles were destroyed, seventeen people were kidnapped, and seventeen others were killed. Among the dead were Bello Damna, the earnest and hammer-fond driver who had carried us safely over so many muddy roads and thorny fields during our early years in Kolofata; Madi Talba, Amadou Ali's reliable brother-in-law who had secreted us out of town that evening four months earlier when there was fear that Boko Haram would get to us first; Moussa, Ali's faithful housekeeper and cook who had served us our first plate of rice and red sauce and who had broken to us as gently as he could the news of 9/11; Issa Plata, one of our most senior nurses; and Amadou Ali's younger brother, Alhadji Malloum.

The attack was the beginning of years of torment for our town and for many other towns along Cameroon's border with northeastern Nigeria. Electricity went off shortly before the Kolofata attack and this time did not come back on. The flow of water stopped completely. Schools and health centers closed. A climate of fear and horror prevailed.

No one knows the exact tally of people killed by Boko Haram or by governments' attempts to corral the group, but estimates put it in the tens of thousands. The number of displaced people is now approaching three million. Houses, shops, and schools have been burned. Villages have been obliterated. Children have been gunned down in their sleep. Thousands of girls and women have been abducted from their homes in Nigeria and neighboring countries and used as sex slaves. By late 2015, increased pressure on Boko Haram militia resulted in kidnapped girls in suicide vests becoming the weapon of choice. In Kolofata alone, terrorist violence has injured 765 people, 526 of them fatally.

Maybe someday we will know if this calamity has been about anything more than the manipulation of populations to create chaos, or if the intended financial and political gain was ever meant to benefit more than a small coterie of individuals, but right now, neither appears to be the case.

The terrorist leaders would like the world to believe that their actions are expressions of piety and obedience to God's will. Yet they know they have commandeered religion and use it no differently than they use opioids, without enlightenment or restraint, to numb minds and induce desperate dependency. They prey on people who are appallingly poor, uneducated, and illiterate but who, in spite of all that, are hopeful that life even for them can be better than it is.

During this reign of terror, the hospital in Kolofata has not shut its doors. Some staff have died and others have left, but enough have remained to continue to offer succor to all who come through our gates. They vaccinate the healthy, treat the sick, deliver babies, mend the injured, and wait.

I, too, wait. I was able to return to Cameroon at the end of 2015, but going as far as Kolofata could not be attempted without putting myself and anyone with me in danger. Occasionally I can get through on the telephone to the chief or other elders of Kolofata. When I ask them what they think about my coming back, they answer hopefully every time: "Soon, soon, maybe two months." So I am waiting these two months, again, and again, and again.

DR. ELLEN EINTERZ has spent most of her life in rural West and Central Africa. After two years as a Peace Corps volunteer in Niger in the mid-1970s, she directed a Catholic mission hospital in Benue State, Nigeria. She moved to northern Cameroon in 1990 and remained for twenty-four years, building and leading a district hospital and public health service. She was medical coordinator of an Ebola Treatment Unit in Liberia during the epidemic of 2014–2015, and she is presently working in Indianapolis, Indiana, with refugees newly arrived from war-torn countries. She is affiliated with Indiana University School of Medicine and Indiana University Fairbanks School of Public Health in Indianapolis.

CPSIA information can be obtained
at www.ICGtesting.com
Printed in the USA
BVHW08s1014190618
519430BV00016B/576/P